# RELEASING THE
# COMPASSION

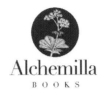

## Alchemilla
### B O O K S

Published in the UK in 2021 by Annie Dransfield
Copyright © Annie Dransfield 2021
Annie Dransfield has asserted her right under
the Copyright, Designs and Patents Act, 1988,
to be identified as the author of this work.

For permission requests contact authorannied54@gmail.com

Paperback    ISBN 978-1-9196063-0-9
eBook        ISBN 978-1-9196063-1-6

Cover design and typeset by SpiffingCovers.com

# RELEASING THE
# COMPASSION

⸺◦⊗◦⸺

## ANNIE DRANSFIELD

An exposé of the threat that is binding the hands
of our community's most needed carers

# Contents and How to Use this Book

**Acknowledgements**

**About the Author**

**Preface**

**Get Real**

**Chapter 1** - History of Caring

**Chapter 2** - What Is a Social Injustice?

**Chapter 3** - Do I Look Invisible?

**Chapter 4** - A Carer's Analogy

**Chapter 5** - Carers' Qualities and Skills

**Chapter 6** - Who Cares Anyway?

- Dissociation by Family and Friends
- Who Cares for the Carer?
- Coping Strategies

## Chapter 7 - Engaging with Agencies – Lived Experiences

Health and Social Care
- Health and Social Care
- Working Between and Across Government Departments
- Local Authority
- Care Homes
- Corporate Business

*There are eleven Lived Experiences in Chapter 7*
*Each of the titles above include a:*

- A Lived Experience
- Personal Reflection for Discussion
- There's a Frog in the Basement – Unexpected incidents that have to be dealt with as soon as possible
- What Now? – One problem follows another
- Discussion Points

## Chapter 8 - A Vision of Life and Caring in 2050

## Chapter 9 - Activities

## Gallery

## References

**Key Features**

- To guide and give encouragement to carers when faced with a social injustice
- To use as a learning resource in business/training/ healthcare/support groups/community projects
- To raise awareness and encourage private sectors and corporate business to reflect on their practice
- To discuss and think about how a carer's life can be improved by historical events

**How to use this book in Chapter 7**

*Chapter 7 talks about engaging with agencies and includes Lived Experiences in all of the categories below:*

- Health and Social Care
- Working Between and Across Government Departments
- Local Authority
- Care Homes
- Corporate Business

**There are eleven Lived Experiences in Chapter 7**

- Lived Experience 1 Health and Social Care Deprivation of Oxygen at Birth
- Lived Experience 2 Health and Social Care Hemiplegia
- Lived Experience 3 Health and Social Care Injury to the Brain
- Lived Experience 4 Health and Social Care Managing a Disability

- Lived Experience 5 Health and Social Care Mental Health
- Lived Experience 6 Working Between and Across Government Departments Legal Roles and Finances
- Lived Experience 7 Working Between and Across Government Departments Direct Payments
- Lived Experience 8 Local Authority Talks about Finances and Care Homes
- Lived Experience 9 What is it Really Like Being a Relative for a Loved One in a Care Home
- Lived Experience 10 Mobile Phones
- Lived Experience 11 Better Banking for Carers

**After each of the Lived Experiences there is:**

- Personal Reflection
- There's a Frog in the Basement – Unexpected incidents that have to be dealt with as soon as possible
- What Now? – One problem follows another
- Discussion Points

**The content in this book can be used for the following:**

- Training and discussion purposes in business, health and social care.
- Carer support groups and community projects related to caring, in addition to role playing and theatrical companies who deal with mental health.

**Learning Outcomes:**

- What are the key points in these carer's experiences?
- What worked well?
- What do we need to do?
- What have you learnt from these experiences?
- How can the situations be improved?

## Chapter 9: Activities for Training Purposes.

*There are a total of eight Activities*

- Activity 1: The Perceptual Table – The way in which something is regarded, understood or interpreted
- Activity 2: Moral Values, Social Skills and Communication
- Activity 3: Who's Knocking on my Door?
- Activity 4: Role Play
- Activity 5: Now That's What I call Care Share
- Activity 6: Care Share – Let's keep a sense of humour
- Activity 7: Talk About Words
- Activity 8: Talk, Listen, Respond

# Acknowledgements

First and foremost to my wonderful, caring, loving and sensitive son, without whom, despite his disabilities and the injustices we have faced together in our journey to date, this book would never have been written.

To my wonderful husband Peter who has supported me with numerous coffees, love and words of wisdom whilst shut away in my office writing.

Many thanks to my very supportive friends and colleagues at the University of Leeds in the School of Healthcare especially Dr Elaine McNichol and Dr Gary Morris for their outstanding mentorship, encouragement and moral support.

To my very special friends David Proudlove, former Chair of the Carers UK, Leeds Branch, and Dee, his lovely wife, for their wonderful sense of humour and support. To all my friends at Carers UK Leeds Branch, particularly Val Hewison, Chief Executive Officer, who has dedicated her life to supporting carers, our thumbs are worn out with all the texting during this pandemic, and to all her hard-working, and just as dedicated, staff, volunteers and carers.

For all the staff I have worked with at Carers UK London including Imelda, Helena, Madeline, David, Michael, Matt,

Gavin, Fern and all other former staff who supported me with Better Banking for Carers along with Dame Philippa Russell and my MP, Stuart Andrew, who was just as passionate about my campaign as I was.

To Kauser, Brian and Ann for their contributions to this book and to all my fellow carers.

I sincerely thank Mick Ward, Ian Brooke Mawson and Bridget McGuire of Adult Social Services, Leeds City Council and members of the strategy group for caring about carers.

To the wonderful publishing team at SpiffingCovers who have been great to work with and so helpful and supportive.

My thanks to Chris Butler CEO of the Leeds and York Partnership Foundation Trust and all staff who I worked with for many years in my role of Carer Governor for the Trust. This includes a special note of thanks to Dr Diss and his team at the Assertive Outreach Team for all their outstanding help and support over the years and, last but not least, a special and sincere thanks to all my readers. All the experiences depicted in this book are true, names, places and relationships have been changed to protect identity.

# About the Author

Born and brought up in Yorkshire, Annie wrote her first radio play whilst at secondary school. After leaving school, one of her short children's stories was also broadcast on radio. Her love of English, speech, drama and writing has been a big part of her life writing scripts for theatre, and co-author for academic magazines on carer involvement. She has written, produced, directed and performed in numerous theatre productions for Leeds Art Theatre.

Following on from her many years working for the health service as a middle manager, Annie went to college where she trained and passed the Guildhall Speech and Drama exams, going on to train as a qualified lecturer in further education where she taught arts and entertainment and special educational needs drama, dance and movement. On being offered and accepting a post teaching drama and performing arts at a boarding school, she produced many musicals with the junior and senior classes in addition to drama therapy with the Special Educational Needs Department of the school. Annie unfortunately decided to retire very early in order to look after her son full-time, therefore becoming an unpaid carer.

Her years of experience in caring took her into a different realm of teaching as a visiting lecturer in the School of Healthcare at the University of Leeds, speaking to student nurses and social workers on all aspects of caring in addition to her involvement in research programmes and interviewing students from a carer's perspective and special carer events.

As a carer member of the Adult Social Services, Annie wrote the foreword for the launch of the Carers Strategy Implementation Group magazine in addition to being a governor for the Leeds and York Partnership Foundation Trust and Chair of several Patient Participation Forums.

Public speaking on all aspects of caring in mental health has played a great part in Annie's life in which she had the privilege of being one of the speakers in a conference on democratic professionalism in addition to organisations such as BUPA, Samaritans Disabled Centre, carers groups, conferences and events.

As a governor of the Leeds York and Partnership Foundation Trust, Annie, with Chief Executive Chris Butler, took part in a radio interview on unpaid carers and caring. The highlights in her caring life were when she was invited to the BBC Television Studios in Manchester to speak about sandwich caring, followed by several radio interviews, in addition to her Better Banking for Carers campaign.

Annie, now a former trustee for Carers UK and governor for the Leeds York and Partnership Foundation Trust, is still an active member of the trust's Carers Steering Group.

Awards: Carer of the Year Award, Carer Champions Award, High Sheriff Award

# Preface

Have you ever been faced with a situation where you have had to make a complaint and, in doing so, you find the other party saying one thing when it suits their instant purpose, and then the opposite when it suits a later purpose, living in hope that we will never detect the inconsistencies?

This is duplicitous behaviour, sneaky and deceitful. Unfortunately, I have come across this too many times in my life as a carer, and from listening to other carers' predicaments they have experienced much the same.

Social injustices in caring is the main theme of this book, and its primary aim is designed with a view to, by virtue of the genuine, lived experiences depicted, being a useful resource. I write this practical, realistic and no-nonsense account as a layperson, not from an academic angle, however, it is conducive to various businesses and organisations, corporate or private, in addition to education, including university lecturers and students in health and social care, mental health and, of course, carers' support groups.

The purpose of accentuating my lived experiences in this book is to raise awareness of problems that could, and do, arise and how I dealt with them. I hope that these will give carers some support in their own situations. At the same time, my experiences endeavour to help carers speak out with confidence, to persevere, challenge, question and gather facts, and, if nothing else, to know that you are not alone.

In the carer's calendar, there is not a day goes by, for some of us, without us having to face some barrier with public services and/ or external agencies who do not understand the complexities of caring. If all the services carers have to deal with for their loved ones are provided efficiently and correctly this makes a carer's job much easier; if the service user is happy then so is the carer and vice versa.

By highlighting the predicaments and unjust incidents that unpaid carers frequently face in everyday life, the lived experiences are intended to act as a resource for carers and professionals in the hope that they will inspire and positively ignite discussion and debate amongst those who aspire to use this as a useful means to accompany one's learning and outcomes.

It is envisaged that, from the content of this material, one will look more deeply into the practical issues that carers and their loved ones are faced with in order to gain more of an insight into how these may affect them and what we can all do differently that will help improve the life of an unpaid carer.

Having been involved in many patient and public involvement groups over a considerable number of years, it is apparent from the ideas and suggestions put forward by carers and service users and put into practice by professionals, that there is no doubt that the input of these lived experiences are a valuable and priceless resource, instrumental to all organisations that deal with the public along with health care professionals, in terms of listening to ideas and suggestions from a carer's perspective.

As well as being carers, we are also customers and patients that use the same services as everyone else. However, we are customers with an extremely demanding and important role in society that not only saves the government billions of pounds, but that can give invaluable, genuine and original input into many areas of business, education and health care.

Be it government departments, private sectors or external organisations, from my personal lived experiences, they require essential, not just desirable, change to meet the needs of carers and their loved ones. When professionals are seen to be genuinely helping carers with their queries, practical needs, services and products, I have no doubt that their reputation will be enhanced, in addition to others who may benefit financially, in other words, a bank with good customer service which is carer and service user-friendly is highly likely to increase its customers.

Unfortunately, external organisations, those who are not in the health care sector, seem reluctant to involve carers which is regrettable, as very often their input can be a powerful resource in being able to see what professionals may not, and this could be the very asset that contributes towards innovation and implementing new, purposeful and an uncomplicated provision of services.

Involve carers who are using your services and include them in contributing to proposed changes which could affect the way they are caring for a loved one, this includes discussions, planning, reviewing and developing services.

In many aspects, where staff training is concerned, in order to support their more vulnerable customers and carers, training is imperative and just as essential as the services and products one provides, therefore, with an organisation's expertise, businesses can turn negative, and sometimes very unpleasant, situations into much more positive ones to support their more vulnerable customers and carers and could do no worse than to revisit and appraise their own approach by way of staff training, thinking, attitude and practice from a practical, moral and social angle. This may mean adapting policies, procedures and systems that fit and meet the needs of the carer and not the other way round.

External agencies often send emails inviting people to give feedback, however it is highly unlikely that carers get invitations to give face-to-face feedback to a company when using them on behalf of their loved ones.

For example, as lasting power of attorney (LPA) for my mother, I get emails from the bank. These pop up on the screen, and the first thing I read is '*Hi Rose, tell us how we are doing*'. At the age of ninety-three, and suffering with dementia and other physical and mental health difficulties, she of course is not going to respond. I would, but I don't. Why? For the simple reason feedback forms such as this do not include a section to enable the carer to give comments. If there was I would be sending an email saying '*Hi Bank, you know I am an LPA for my mother Rose, please include both of our names, or just mine, on this email*'.

When I receive surveys or similar from social services, Carers UK or Carers Leeds, they are specifically designed for the carer and, on some, for the service users to complete. This is good practice. NHS England state that they are committed to ensuring that public and patients are at the centre of how they shape health care services.

Credit where credit is due as far as external agencies go, an established provider of gas and electric with the name British in it, in my experience, does just this. Their emails acknowledge both me and my son. This is definitely good practice, because it tells me that they recognise I am a carer and that I am responsible for my son's accounts, thereby treating him as an individual who they also recognise as a service user.

Carer involvement is a crucial and constructive element in any part of research and design, in this case underpinned by the written and verbal feedback of student nurses and social workers in the School of Healthcare at the University of Leeds. It includes evidence on how a carer's expertise has enhanced and supported the students' learning of their chosen profession, with lecturers and students agreeing that highlighting the real complexities of a carer's life are an asset to their learning.

From the many teaching sessions I have had the privilege and pleasure of speaking at, over a number of years at Leeds University in the School of Healthcare, I illustrate a few of the feedback statements taken from various classes of student mental health nurses. Below, I refer to a few from the one hundred and twenty-four feedback sheets I received over a period of six sessions.

- How did you feel listening to Annie's experiences?

- What have you learnt about the caring role and day-to-day experience of carers?
- How will this help you in the future when in practice?

*It is a very hard and demanding role which you never get a break from, along with being physically, emotionally and psychologically drained.*

*Involve carers as much as possible.*

*This talk helped me understand the responsibilities of a carer and that this should be acknowledged when caring for a service user.*

*The amount on unseen work that is done by carers.*

*I felt inspired by listening to Annie's day-to-day experience and it also raised awareness of the lack of support for carers in some areas.*

*I will vow to continue to include family in the care of service users when in practice.*

*It will help me to understand what carers are going through and that they are people as well.*

*I will involve and engage with carers, be empathic and listen actively to the carer's concerns.*

*It was a very informative talk hearing about the many aspects of caring and it gave me a new appreciation of the difficulties in caring.*

*Touching and emotional.*

*I could really feel the emotion in her speech and how passionate she was about making changes.*

I became a carer in the 1970s for my son, Jay, who was born with a deprivation of oxygen resulting in him being diagnosed with special needs and cerebral palsy; consequently the majority of his early years were spent attending hospital, at least several times a week.

As he became older, due to the complications at birth, he was diagnosed with an acute mental health problem. In those days, I was what we now call a 'hidden carer'. I still care for my son and all aspects of his life, including managing his finances and paperwork as his deputy through a Court of Protection order.

Although unbelievable, it soon became apparent that the injustices I faced as a carer for Jay were just as prevalent for my parents as well, albeit in different scenarios. My father passed away after suffering many years of severe Alzheimer's and cancer, whilst my mother, who had a stroke and as a consequence dementia and Alzheimer's, is still living.

Like all carers, our responsibilities and concerns are part of our caring territory and daily contemplation, however, throw into the carer's pot a multitude of complex issues, major problems and minor irritations, mix with the extensive, agonising and exasperating mishandling of our discontent, the narrow-mindedness from individuals who blank, overlook or presume they know better, and we are left with an overflowing, half-baked boiling pot with more than enough issues to drive us up the wall.

Throughout all my years of caring, I have seen services that have developed for the better, who demonstrate already implemented, exemplary practice, in terms of staff attitude, services provided, along with support, compassion and understanding towards the carer. However, I still become frustrated and disillusioned by other services at the lack of development in systems, policies and procedures which can completely overlook the carer's role. The practical and soul-stirring difficulties we have to deal with affect us physically, emotionally, psychologically, spiritually and socially, when common sense, logic, understanding, support and recognition are not forthcoming by some professionals and non-carers.

The needs of your loved one will be varied and many, in terms of their physical and/ or mental health difficulties, however, the basic elements of a person's day-to-day lifestyle are common to us all, so as carers we are not only trying to look after our own basic needs but that of our loved ones as well.

My lived experiences aim to underpin all the issues I, and other carers, deal with (in my case my son and parents) that you might well be dealing with for your loved one/s or, at least, may recognise in your carer's role.

My book, *Releasing the Compassion*, goes behind the scenes to reveal what really happens backstage. What are the realities of dealing with incidents in a carer's life? I am revealing true events that have happened to me and the impact that other people's careless and thoughtless words and actions have on the carer and their loved one.

Problems and injustices all generate paperwork, telephone

calls, visits, meetings, time and money. They all demand liaising with other people in various ways according to the nature of the issue/s. We have to be very careful and accurate in the way we communicate, for example by letter, email and phone. We have to choose our words carefully, and this is very difficult to do sometimes when, deep inside our hearts, we are upset, stressed, angry and annoyed.

If we communicate by phone, we have to try to keep 'a lid on it' about how we truly feel, keep our voice calm and not indicate frustration or the gradual loss of temper as the call progresses, or not, as the case may be.

Face-to-face meetings are better because we can read other people's body language, but it does not alleviate the sheer frustration of not being listened to. Even more so when our legitimate complaint is trivialised, or another version of events given, along with issues being marginalised and the truth twisted, or ignored altogether. All of these involve the recipient of the complaint to listen and address the issues put before them; they all necessitate both parties relying on knowledge, wisdom, understanding, attitude, common sense, logic and compassion, to name but a few.

For the carer, I have no doubt that they will be familiar with many of the issues in the Lived Experiences that are featured, along with the injustices I have faced and how I dealt with them and, in doing this, I sincerely hope they will help you, the carer, if ever subjected to similar ones.

Life for any person brings its problems, yet experiencing these problems stood in carers' shoes, a simple task can turn into a nightmare. I know, because I have had a superabundance of them to deal with, and from the hundreds of carers I have met, and still know over forty plus years, they have as well. Why do our experiences end up stressing us out emotionally and, at the same time, practically, giving us copious amounts of paperwork to deal with? Why does it have to be like this?

Sometimes, as we go about our daily routine of: shopping, banking, making appointments with GPs, ordering and collecting medication, getting a taxi to the hospital, seeing the consultant, acting as a power of attorney, dealing with the DWP, visiting a loved one in the care home and sorting out issues with social services, injustices can, and regularly do, occur and the list is immeasurable. Therefore life, due to other people's ineptitude, can be a minor hindrance, a stumbling block that manifests itself into a massive boulder, a great pain in the neck, or a major source of disruption and trouble. How do we deal with unsatisfactory and unacceptable complications and disagreements?

At home, and aside from all the external issues, we just get on with life, with family and friends, to the best of our ability and time available. Family visits, meals together, chatter about the present and past, happy memories of looking through old photos from times gone by that allow us to laugh at fashions, transport, places and people, along with the traditions and celebrations of special occasions, all give us reason to share our different faiths, open presents, watch fireworks and play on the beach among many other things.

I think myself incredibly fortunate to have had a very happy childhood brought up in a working-class background full of laughter, and sometimes tears, and with the freedom to play out safely.

Now as a superannuitant (well, it sounds better than old fogey doesn't it?), as a family, we are now the ones who instigate, encourage and stimulate parents with the days of yesteryear as they reach their elderly years. My dad was independent till Alzheimer's took hold and, although ageing, my dad was always a positive person and made us laugh constantly, whilst my mum was a little more serious and tended to worry more. From the comical to the alarming and worrying predicaments before and after my parent's elderly years took their toll, Dad made us laugh, intentionally and unintentionally. One of the unintentional incidents was when my parents were out shopping together. They stopped to look at the men's and ladies' clothes in a shop window and then decided to go in and have a look around.

After half an hour or so, Mum, armed with the cardigan and other few bits and pieces she needed, looked around for Dad and could not see him anywhere. She thought he was probably chatting to someone he knew, or didn't know, as he was the type of person who would make casual conversation with others whilst waiting for Mum.

Having paid for her goods, Mum went outside, but Dad was nowhere to be seen. She stood by the shop window waiting, and wondering where on earth he had got to, when suddenly she heard a loud tapping on the glass behind her. When she turned around, she saw Dad on his knees, on the floor of the display window, hanging on to one of the mannequins, looking out at her.

Mum was not pleased and said tight-lipped, "What the hell are you doing in there?"

His muffled reply, "I fell."

The times that family have fun and laugh together are precious moments that all too soon become treasured memories. When they became ill, we cared regularly from a distance and one day travelled the one hundred and sixty-mile round trip to check on them, after I had tried to contact them by phone and could not get any answer which was very unusual.

When we got to their home, the double gates were closed and all was quiet, now I was really bothered. I knocked on the door. Mum answered it with a surprised look on her face.

"What are you doing here?" she said.

I said, "Just passing by, so thought we would call in."

"Why, where have you been?"

"We haven't been anywhere. I have been trying to get you on the phone most of the day, and you weren't answering; we were so worried about you both and wondered if you were alright."

"The phone's not rung here. Must be something wrong with it."

On inspection, we found that Dad had unplugged the phone instead of unplugging the vacuum.

When we got back home, tired but relieved that all was well

with my parents, we went to up to bed. I was too tired to read and just lay there for a few minutes relaxing, when my husband broke the silence by talking to himself.

"What did you say?"

He said, "I was just asking myself what day is it, and when I have to take this tablet, and it says on the packet *NOW*. That's clever isn't it, only I realised that I was reading, *MON*, the day of the week on the packet, upside down."

Tired, anxious, confused, exhausted, and living on Costas and takeaways is all part of life for the carer, particularly when your loved ones go into hospital. I sat there filling in the form called 'This is me' for patients with Alzheimer's. I have lost count of how many of these I have completed, in terms of conveying all the relevant details about Dad, in order to help the staff.

When we visited the following day, he had been moved to another ward, and did the 'This is me' form go with him? No, so I had to fill another one in. Why do I have to repeat this task again? It is taking away precious visiting time with my lovely dad. At one time, fit and healthy physically and mentally, Dad was in the kitchen and all of us sat talking to Mum in the lounge after tea. *Clatter, bang, clatter, bang, clatter, clatter, crash.*

"What's all the noise?" I exclaimed.

"It's only your dad doing the washing up. No wonder I've not got any pots left."

Then one day Mum had a stroke. Stabilised now, but still very ill and confused, we were sat with her as she lay in bed. The room she was in was on the top floor of the building, it had a window at the back of her bedhead and a large window opposite her looking into the corridor of the ward.

"I didn't sleep well last night," she said. We asked why that was. "There was a little boy in the room, and he was stood on that windowsill. He had his little hands and face pressed to the window looking out into the corridor. Poor, little thing was crying and saying he wanted to be with his mummy at the party, then all these little coloured birds flew on to the sill with him." We were brought back to reality, when my husband saw a red kite gliding in the sky outside.

Back at the hospital with Dad, they were doing an assessment and the nurse who was asking him questions held up a large, laminated, coloured poster full of small, square photos of various examples of stools/motions.

"Can you tell me, Edward, which one is most like yours?"

It was like a question you would get on the mobile from a buzz quiz: "From the list below, which is unlike any of the others?"

Dad pondered the images for a while before saying, "Well, there's that many, I don't know which one to choose."

"You don't choose one, Dad; you say which one is like yours when you go to the loo for a poo." This was one question I certainly could not help answer for him.

"Okay," said the nurse, "we will move to the next question. How is your health generally?"

"Well, I don't smoke, I don't drink, and I don't have sex; pretty good I would say." He always saw the bright side of life, always a joke or two to tell and always with a twinkle in his eyes.

After Mum had her stroke, she took ill again some months later suffering with severe psychosis, acute delirium and hallucinations. She was dreadfully upset, agitated and frightened. As we sat in the waiting room of A & E, she told us about the dangerous, threatening, wild animals that she could see in the waiting room with us.

"One of them is over there, look." They were predatory, savage animals in the form of wild dogs. Her expression changed to one of utter disgust, as she wrinkled her nose up and said, "It's doing its mess all over the floor." I am no stranger to witnessing psychosis but even this alarmed and chilled me to the bone.

I had texted my lovely friend Val, the CEO of Carers Leeds, on her mobile, to tell her where we were and what was happening. "*Oh God,*" I punched out rapidly on my phone. "*This is terrible.*" For the duration of our waiting time with Mum in this turbulent state, Val selflessly, relentlessly and compassionately kept me going with a continuous stream of supportive, encouraging and comforting words, even offering to come over to the hospital, which I would not even contemplate, as it was now so late into the evening.

My mother was admitted to the hospital, where she stayed for six weeks. We visited every day and each visit was the same. The unwelcome, untamed, wild dogs, rats, birds and cats continued to petrify her. She smelt their putrid smells and heard their howling, squeaks, yowling and cawing. The bleak and repulsive world she was living in, at this moment in time, made her irritable, irrational, scathing and argumentative, to which we were on the receiving end again, as we arrived for another visit.

I sat down, and she said to me, "What have you come for?"

"We've come to see how you are, Mum."

"Well, you shouldn't be here, not in that state."

"What do you mean, Mum? I'm okay."

"No, you're not; you shouldn't be out looking like that."

Okay, I know I'm not in the league of a model, but hey, beauty is in the eye of the beholder.

"Why, what's wrong with me?"

"It's your eyes, there's something wrong with them."

"What's wrong with them?"

"You've got great big, long worms crawling out of them. Go home."

This vision was so convincing, I even put my hands up to my face, touching my eyes, to see if I could feel anything.

The hallucinations obviously greatly disturbed her. She could not bring herself to look at me, as it was upsetting her so much, that we decided to leave the visit that day and go home.

I did not talk very much regarding my worries and concerns about Jay to my parents. Of course, they knew the background of what had happened to Jay, but the time, in his teens, when he went with a friend to a 'music in the park' festival had me worrying if he was going to be alright. We had always said to call us, no matter what time of the day or night, if he needed us. In the early hours of the morning, we had that call. Jay and his friend had lost each other, so Jay had decided to make his way home, but he'd got lost. We told him to stay where he was, and we would come for him. We found him near a main road, and he had managed to get covered in mud. He was just scared, confused and lost.

My life in caring has given me the opportunity to meet some wonderful people who demonstrate innovation, flair, aptitude, compassion, empathy and determination to make positive changes, so like them, I strive to do my utmost in challenging unfairness and resolving injustices in caring. Your decision to accompany me in this true and turbulent life, as an unpaid carer with its problems, difficulties and unplanned issues cropping up along the way, is very much appreciated.

*Releasing the Compassion* conveys many lived experiences, trials and tribulations of an unpaid carer's role, it highlights the endeavours to right the wrongs and to reiterate the rights of carers, and the importance to speak out and establish our expertise.

You may decide to read it for no other reason than to discover what has gone wrong for me, and how I dealt with it, but I also hope it can be used purposefully in practice, training and discussion to raise awareness of the unrevealed, underlying and unpredicted populace of the carer's landscape.

On behalf of all carers present and future, let us hope that this book will bring back our identity as individuals and be genuinely recognised as carers because, when all said and done, we are the experts.

*Psychiatric Bulletin 2008, Involving Service Users and Carers in Psychiatric Education and Training: What do trainees think? The National Service Framework for Mental Health states that 'service users and carers should be involved in planning, providing and evaluating training for all healthcare professionals' [Department of Health 1999]. In 2004 the Royal College of Psychiatrists committed to increasing involvement of service users and carers throughout psychiatric education. This has been mandatory since June 2005.*

# GET REAL

The world and his wife always have a solution or think they have.

Many carers could possibly be looking after other sons, daughters, grandchildren, nieces, nephews, parents, young children, or a young, working age adult because of mental and/or physical health disabilities. In addition, there are carers who may have another adult in the same family who has an addiction maybe to alcohol, drugs or gambling. Whatever the existing conditions, all of these perplexities impact considerably on the carer. But the question is how do we deal with it?

It's easy for an individual, who is not in any of these situations, to give their opinion and tell us what they would do, but unless they can really put themselves into a carer's world, if they can really show genuine understanding and concern towards a situation, it really does not help, it becomes just another frustrating conversation. GET REAL. I wonder how many times carers have uttered these words.

**GET REAL**

You're making this up – Well actually, I am not

**Reactions:**

I can't believe it really happened like that – Well, it did

Do you think it would be useful if...? – No, it wouldn't

**Attitudes:**

I wouldn't have my lad coming home drunk every night... – Well, he's not your lad. Words just roll off the tongue; it's much harder to put into practice

No way! – Move house

**Approaches:**

Tell him to just go – It is not that simple when they need help

Throw him out – And then where does he go? Out on the streets? This makes the situation worse, because he is not able to get any help and support for the family

**Shock Horror:**

Can't she do it herself? – It's difficult for her and she needs help

Do you think it would be useful if...? – No, it wouldn't

**Embarrassing:**

Have you tried...? – No, I have not, because in my situation that would not be appropriate and, in any case, do you think I have not already thought of that?

How do you really feel? – Do you really want to know?

**Best intentions:**

He/she wouldn't be on drugs if they were mine – It can happen to anyone

Stop giving him money – I don't any more, he earns his own

If I were you... – Well, you're not

**Neighbour:**

"I've reported him for playing music so loudly." – "I am really sorry about that, I'll tell him to turn it down. I don't know if you are aware, but he does have special needs." – "Tough, that's your problem." I was appalled by this neighbour's attitude.

**Mental health:**

A person displaying retarded catatonia may stare into space, not knowing that they may actually be staring at another person, and stare while in deep thought. This happened to Jay when he called into the local pub for a drink (1 pint). He went into a catatonic state whilst sat down listening to his music on his headphones, minding his own business, when some idiot thought he was staring at them, so he just went across to my son and beat him up. My son left the building and went home, however, his friends went up to the young man and told him about my son's condition, they were appalled at what he had done and the landlord gave the naïve lad his marching orders.

I wanted to call the police, but Jay said not to. When he went to the pub a few days later to see his friends, the lad who had laid into him was in there too. Jay sat down to talk to his friends, and the other lad came over to him.

He offered his hand and said, "I'm really sorry about the other day, I'd had a bit to drink." Jay accepted his apology and the lad bought him a drink.

**Arrested:**

Carer: "My niece has just been arrested for taking weed, she was with a load of her friends in somebody's flat when it got raided, and now she is in the police station."

Neighbour: "Best place for her then, and tell your sister to kick her out."

Carer: "That is not the answer, I want to help them."

## Julie and her family

The phone rang. Julie answered it.

"Hello," the voice at the other end said. "Could I speak to Mrs Baines please?"

"Speaking," said Julie.

"It's the secretary at St Peter's Hospital, just wanted to confirm some details on your mum, Mrs Waring's form. I believe she was admitted to hospital yesterday, with a blood clot on her leg."

"Yes, that's right. Is she okay?" Squeals rang out from Jason, sobs from Kelly and banging doors from both, then laughing and yelling. "Can you hold on a moment please?" Julie said, as she turned her attention back to the kids. "Pack that noise in now and calm down, I'm trying to talk to someone on the phone." Back to the caller, "Sorry about that. What were you saying?"

As Julie flipped the lid shut on her smartphone, she suddenly spotted her eldest offspring in the garden, peering through the window, face pressed to the smeary pane from the mucky handprints of the kids. Karl was shouting about something, which made absolutely no sense at all, obviously intoxicated and still with a bottle in his hand and it wasn't milk.

"Oh, for goodness' sake," she said out loud, "I can do without him at the moment."

"Mam, Mam, are you there?" *Bang, bang,* on the pane of glass with his hand, then changing to the metal bit of his dogs lead, *clunk, chink, clunk.*

"Stop banging on that bloody window and just come through the door, or, better still, stay out there till you've calmed down and shut up."

"Mam," shouts Karl.

"What, what do you want now, Karl?"

"Can you lend me a tenner, please? I ain't got no benefit till next week, and I need some pet food."

"How many times have I told you, I cannot keep giving you money?"

Karl, swaying a little, walked into the house. "I know, but I really need it because I can't feed Bassy tonight."

"Well, you shouldn't have got the flaming dog in the first place, when you can barely look after yourself."

"Please, Mum."

From anger, frustration and the sheer distress that her son was like this, the hopelessness of it all, Julie grabbed her bag and wrenched out her purse.

"Mam?"

"What now?"

"Can you make it twenty? It'll just give me that bit extra to get some food as well."

"Food, as in a six-pack you mean. For goodness' sake, Karl, this is typical of you. Give an inch and you want a yard. This is it now, twenty quid. Don't you dare ask for any more, because you are not getting it, got it?"

"Yes, suppose so. Where's our Linda?" Karl asked.

"She's over at her friends doing homework, and don't even think about asking her for her pocket money."

"Is Robby okay?"

"He's at the day centre today with his care worker, as well you should know. I get two days' respite a week, Karl, and it would be good if you could lend a hand sometime, but that will never happen will it, because you always end up upsetting him."

"We must never upset Robby, must we?"

"Just go home, Karl."

When the kids were in bed reading and Robby had been bathed and fed and was now listening to his music in his room, Mike and Julie finally sat down. They had been married a long time, and Mike was her pillar of strength.

"How's your day been, Julie?" Mike asked.

"Well, it was going okay until the kids got home from school, as usual bickering, arguing, and running around when the hospital rang. I could hardly hear myself think. They wanted some details on Mum, then, to top it all, Karl showed up."

"I guess he wanted money to feed Bassy."

"Yes, he did," replied Julie, "and did you know that his dog, a basenji, is just like a cat; good hunters, so I am informed. They have a stubborn streak, just like Karl, they know commands, but whether they adhere to them or not depends on how they feel, just like Karl. He was brought up to know good from bad, but he goes his own way. Like master, like dog. I am led to believe that this particular breed of dog is barkless, so it's quiet. That is the only thing he does not have in common with it."

The noise from all the laughing and running around was an indication that Jason and Kelly had become fed up with reading. Julie got up to go and speak to them.

"It's alright, I'll go," said Mike. He found them both chucking crisps at each other. "Right, that's it. Get back into bed, and I'll take those crisps. You shouldn't have them up here, anyway. Lights out, and no more noise." Kelly got back into bed, and Jason went back to his room. "Goodnight, you two."

"Night, Dad."

As he walked back into the room, he said to Julie, "Right, they should go to sleep now, but think the carpet will need a vac tomorrow."

"Thank goodness I have a night off from the chippy tonight; I could do with an early night." The children are Julie's grandchildren, her daughter passed away at a young age with cancer.

Carers lives, whilst being very similar in the fundamentals of caring, are very different when other complex ingredients are thrown into the throng of domesticity. Julie, as always, reacted to the 'emotional blackmail' that Karl demanded of her.

If this were a case study at an academic establishment for student mental health nurses, and/or social workers, we would have time for discussion and debate on a vast amount of material that this scenario throws up. At the end of an hour and half teaching session, possible solutions could be talked about to help each member of the family. If, at the end of the session, a solution is not found immediately it does not matter, it can be continued at some stage for further deliberation.

But LET'S GET REAL, at this particular juncture, there is no time for debate, no time for discussion, because carers have to act immediately when there is a crisis. An option or solution has to be found at the time of a problem, or a crisis. The reasoning behind Julie's decision to hand over the money to her son was out of tiredness, despair, her lack of energy to argue, and because she hates conflict. Just take it and go.

To many people this solution would have been the wrong one, yet emotional blackmail is a threat, and in desperation we give in when perhaps we should not. For some carers this situation is REAL.

As carers, we have to tell it the way it is, but we don't. Why don't we? We often hold back on telling professionals, our friends and family, exactly what our real circumstances are because we fear rejection, alienation, stigma and embarrassment along with a lack of understanding from some people who have not experienced our quandary.

From my experience, I have spoken to people who appear to be kind and empathetic, and then morph into well-meaning do-gooders giving advice, which we know will not work, with an air of superiority, leaving us feeling incompetent and a hopeless case.

If you ever that get that gut feeling, that instinct whenever others respond to your situation out of context, detecting that their interpretation is being twisted to suit their needs and criteria, then follow it.

Don't be afraid to say, "Can we just stop there, because this is what is really happening, this is what really needs to be done." You are the expert after all.

If, on the other hand, we talk to professionals who are seeing carers day in, day out, who know instantly what predicaments we are facing, they can identify the issues and proceed to help with a way forward. These people demonstrate a genuine empathy and understanding in a carer's life.

# CHAPTER 1

# History of Caring

History states that in the mid 19th century, one of the first nurses was Florence Nightingale, that private nursing was taking place in the 1920s and mental health disabilities are mentioned as far back as the Greeks with German psychiatrist Emil Kraepelin (1856-1926) who published a comprehensive system of psychological disorders. Disabilities, meaning: physical and/ or mental health problems, have been existent from medieval times, it follows that numerous illnesses have been with us for centuries and, due to the greatest skills of the physicians and scientists of the era, have resulted in phenomenal progress in medicine for physical and mental health. Monumental leaps in psychiatry, from diagnosis to prognoses, along with medication have brought us where we are today in helping people to cope with their mental health difficulties.

I wonder if, in those days, the carer's role was taken into account in terms of the practicalities of caring, and the carer's mental health and well-being, along with carer's assessments and care plans? I strongly suspect none of these were considered at that time, but it does not mean to say that people did not care and looked after those who needed it. I think we can safely say, for sure, that the one aspect, from history to present day, that has not changed is that of a human being's feelings and emotions.

How do we manage when one moment we are demonstrating compassion and understanding to our loved ones, and the next minute we are crestfallen, defeated and let down for a number of reasons. Why? Is it because practical and financial help is not as readily available as it should be? Or is it because we need more help emotionally? We still hear very negative comments and horror stories, in all aspects of caring, despite the carer's pleas for change, whatever the circumstances, it is not always forthcoming.

In the early days of my caring role, I was asked by my care support worker if I would like to go to a care support group. I wasn't quite sure at first, but a month or so later I decided I would. We met some lovely people at the meeting, who talked about their own experiences in caring and who they cared for, and nearly all the carers who attended retold their journeys of the past and present encounters they'd had to deal with.

Some were indeed very harrowing, despairing, tragic and unhappy, and at the same time a colourful patchwork of humour accompanied them. I sat there listening to these incidents being conveyed with the utmost empathy yet becoming more and more puzzled, disheartened and troubled by the realisation dawning on me that most of these situations did not have a solution or a happy outcome, in terms of getting any immediate, preventative and percipient help from professionals. A problem shared is a problem halved, as the old saying goes, but it is still a problem, and will remain a problem until a solution is found.

Professional, proactive and incredibly supportive are just several of the words that spring to mind to describe our care support worker at that time. We met a few weeks later, after I had been to the support group, and he asked me if I had enjoyed the meeting. I replied that we had met some lovely people there, and it was a pleasant evening along with being able to share their lived experiences, albeit despondent.

"Will you go to the next one?" he asked.

I said I did not think I would, mainly because I found it extremely frustrating listening to other carer's upsetting and various stories without being able to do anything about it.

"However," I said, "if there is a group that can do something more practical and proactive in turning these horror stories into positive ones, I would definitely go to that."

He told me about the Carers Action Group which was about influencing change in mental health run by the facilitator, a lovely lady called Lockie, who enabled carers to help develop services for the people they care for and themselves.

The main aim of the group is to influence change in mental health services throughout Leeds by ensuring all services are appropriate for both service users and carers, the Leeds Mental Health Trust's Carers Team supported this group.

I went along to their next meeting, where I met members who were just as enthusiastic and passionate as I was about mental health and in working together with the professionals in order to look at the many experiences of caring in its holistic format and, in so doing, liaising with professionals in all areas of medical expertise as well as management.

Engagement and involvement are the two key factors in the process of working together, and this aspect has developed immensely over the years in mental health. Carers and service users are invited to be part of discussions with professionals in a range of mental health services, where carers are valued, respected, listened to and their issues addressed.

After some time of being a member, I wrote a working document for the Carers Action Group which listed the services already established within the Leeds Mental Health Trust. Sometimes these services did not always run smoothly, evidenced by carers and service users' experiences, and with this in mind, the negative experience a carer had gone through was discussed and addressed within the Trust's structures and the Carers Action Group worked with services to reduce these negative experiences and achieve positive solutions with them.

In the same document, we had a list of areas where it appeared there was little or no support at all, and again this was devised from the indefensible, poor and disastrous journeys carers had had in all aspects of caring. However, the buck does not just stop with health professionals but with external agencies as well, but that is another chapter.

Taking each of these issues in turn, we aimed to put forward our suggestions and ideas to the Trust about how we could devise a new support mechanism and develop that particular area. In short, the LCAG aimed to turn the horror stories we heard from carers into positive experiences. Already, we had tremendous support from Chris Butler, the chief executive officer at that time of the Leeds Teaching Hospitals Trust (LTHT) with whom we worked closely. We had many meetings with Chris about the goals we would like to achieve, and he approved and supported the document that we presented to him at an open evening event.

It was an exciting time for the LCAG, as we now found ourselves not only the first consultation group, at that time, but now in the process of becoming citywide, with future meetings being held at the Becklin Centre, as opposed to being held at St. Mary's Hospital in Leeds.

<u>Improvement of Services for Service Users and Carers</u>

The Leeds Carers Action Group (LCAG) had a direct link to the Working Age Adult's Service User and Carer Clinical Governance Team which was responsible for improving the quality of services to working age adults with mental health difficulties. This link was through the facilitator of the LCAG who was a staff member of the Leeds and York Partnership Foundation Trust and, as a carer member of the LCAG, I would attend the Clinical Governance meetings with the facilitator.

In order to improve services for carers and service users, an event was held by the Trust which was attended by members of the Leeds Carers Action Group and many other professionals and carers from across the city. It was so encouraging and reassuring to know that our CEO and carers had a common goal.

Having had this event, the CEO asked carer members of the LCAG which three aspects for improvement we would like to start working on.

**Report dated 28th June 2006**

These were:
- Confidentiality including inpatient care
- Crisis management
- External agencies

<u>Confidentiality and Inpatient Care</u>

**Confidentiality:** is an area that springs up and hits you in the face in any situation or circumstances, it is an area which can often stop the carer from caring efficiently and effectively, and certainly one that comes into play in mental health issues where professionals' hands are often tied through government legislation.

However, as carers, we feel that common sense and logic should prevail when a carer is distraught over, say, perhaps an incident, and need their questions answering in an appropriate and reassuring way. The carer asking questions of their loved one is most likely to be the main carer and more often than not involved in their loved one's care on a daily basis.

I myself have been on the receiving end of this very common statement, "I am sorry, I cannot tell you that due to confidentiality". But the silly thing is that Jay had always given his consent for staff to discuss anything with me. We have never had any secrets, and we can talk about anything together, in fact, Jay has always said if I know what is going on I can help him.

Carers know about confidentiality rights and regulations, but I feel that sometimes discretion needs to be exercised in terms of reassuring the carer without breaching the service user's confidentiality rights.

So what happened in my case? Jay was in hospital on a section (of the Mental Health Act), and he had been there a few days. Our care support worker suggested to us that we take ourselves on a short break and unwind, as Jay would be quite safe in the hospital. We sort of hummed and hawed for a while, deliberating about what we should do, when finally, we decided a break would be good, but just for a few days.

We booked a caravan on a tranquil resort; I remember it being very cold, so cold that we had to go and buy a thick duvet to keep us warm at night, and, although I was enjoying the rest, my mind was on Jay. I just kept getting this feeling that all was not well, and I told my husband about it. On the third evening, we went to a restaurant for a meal and, halfway through the main course, my phone rang. It was the hospital to say that Jay had gone.

We abandoned the meal, went back to the caravan, packed our cases, and, in less than an hour, we were back on the road to Leeds. I phoned the hospital as soon as we got home, but Jay was still missing, so we got in the car and went straight up to the hospital.

"Is he back?" I asked.

"No, he isn't."

I asked how he had managed to walk out of the hospital with no one seeing him, but they could not answer that. My husband asked the staff how long they would leave it before informing the police about a missing patient. Jay's health and safety was paramount. They said twenty-four hours. That amount of time had come and gone.

I said, "We are going home, we are going to have a cup of tea, and if I have not had any news by then, we are ringing the police."

Just as we were brewing the tea, the phone went again. It was one of the staff whom we had known for a long time, and she knew Jay really well. She told us that he was with a friend, a girl he had known for a long time. I asked for the girl's number, of course they were not allowed to give out numbers, so she said she would ring her and get Jay to ring me.

Jay rang and said, "What's up, Mum?"

"What's up, Jay? I was worried sick about where you had gone."

"I'm okay. I came home with Cathy to make sure she got home okay." We took Jay back to the hospital, and in a few weeks he was well enough to come home.

**Inpatient Care:** Two of our LCAG members expressed a deep concern on this issue and consequently, with consent, visited a ward and discussed issues of concern with the manger and gave feedback to the group with a comprehensive report.

**Our members' findings were as follows:**

Past experience of visiting wards had always felt uncomfortable, however, after our recent visit and meeting, we were made to feel welcome and felt at ease to ask relevant and equivocal questions. Patients seemed content and the visiting carers were free to chat to patients and staff. Activities in the past seemed sparse, but this visit highlighted more activities with a variety of choice and patients being encouraged to take part; however these activities were still not available on a weekend. Patients are encouraged to comment and contribute on their own treatment. We noted that patients saw doctors three or four times a week, as opposed to just once a week, and although this is a big improvement, they would like to see doctors visiting patients every day, the fact that they don't maybe due to a lack of staff. They said that they were told that the Trust is seeking to maximise self-determination, minimise intrusion in a safe and therapeutic environment and are trying to achieve this through transparency in treatment plans, as well as in communication, and by minimising restrictions upon patients and visitors. Their findings in the report of this particular area, concluded by stating that inpatient care has improved and they felt much more at ease after this meeting.

**Crisis Management**

This service is already up and running, which initially gave tremendous hope to many carers in its early planning stages, but again a service which, through carers' experiences, can be developed even further. Our members on this case stated that they wanted to see carers more involved with the crisis team and, at the moment, there are no carers on the Clinical Governance Team.

They also raised the question of what happens to the person we are caring for after the carer dies. Electronic patient records, that give vital information whenever and wherever a crisis occurs, are vital and they welcomed an initiative that would produce a much more efficient, quicker and higher standard of communication with hospitals and GPs etc.

One of our members met with the manager of the Crisis Resolution Team, at that time, who said that he wants to see more carers involved and was willing to come and give a talk at our meetings, going on to say that care plans are fundamentally important as well as training for all staff in establishing these.

He was also keen to see an electronic patient record system. 'End of Life' workshops were suggested by another professional, in terms of implementing workshops that will inform carers of choices that could be put into place in the event of a demise with one suggestion being to invite a solicitor in to give a talk. The manager informed us, a week or so later, that over the coming months he was going to be working on raising the awareness of carers needs in the Crisis Resolution Service.

**External Agencies**

This third aspect is not one that is primarily related to mental health at the moment, however it is certainly a contributing factor when carers looking after all aspects of a working adult's life have to liaise with third parties i.e. providers of gas, electric, TV licences, water board, telephone companies, banks, building societies and whole host of other providers that demand a carer's attention on a day-to-day or monthly basis of monitoring finances and dealing with correspondence for the person they care for.

Our main aim on this matter is to see, at some point in the future, key workers in organisations, which are not health related, who can communicate with carers and service users in a sensitive and compassionate way, along with answering carers' queries and solving discrepancies in the same manner.

This is about communicating and raising awareness with all agencies, which we as carers deal with on our loved one's behalf, on a regular basis, in terms of paying bills, setting up direct debits, making enquiries and sorting out problems with providers. What we would like to see is a liaison officer in each department who has knowledge and understanding of mental health issues and can deal with our problems directly instead of it being passed from person to person. Much the same as physical disabilities are catered for in and outside of establishments, and rightly so, such as ramps and other disability aids which are provided by them. However, we also need a friendly face, a person who has the ability to deal with our concerns with passion and integrity.

Two health professionals, acting as facilitators in our group, discussed devising a letter we could send to organisations with the suggestion that we need to emphasise the impact that mental ill health, not just on the service user's health but the carer's as well, can have upon a person's ability to deal with things like bills and debt, that carers invariably have to sort out, and it is imperative to have the CEOs and managers from organisations on board to stop these things happening, for example provisions being cut off, ending up in court for not paying credit cards and being evicted because the housing benefit form has not been completed or they cannot pay the rent.

This report, as I said, is from fourteen years ago and, believe it or not, I am still having the same conversations about certain aspects of it, to this day, as I was then.

Let's get real. When is someone going to have a conversation with me about putting these plans into action and employing, or using an existing member of staff, preferably a carer themselves, who knows what we are going through, to help us when we walk into that organisation for help and support?

Leeds Mental Health Trust is to be commended for involving and listening to carers and service users in their discussions and practices, so too would external agencies if they also adopted this method with their customers.

Raising awareness of the work that the Leeds Mental Health Trust supports is a vital part of developing services and, as a carer for many years, the optimum change within the Trust has been to involve carers and service users.

Without the support of the chief executive, the manager of the Carers Development Support Team and public involvement, the CAG's initiatives would never have been given the opportunity to be brought to fruition.

One of our main concerns was to build a much-needed relationship between carers and psychiatrists, which at that time was not as good as it could have been. An example of this was when a psychiatrist, on reviewing a service user's discharge, it was quite clear and obvious to the carers that their son was not well enough to go home; therefore, discharge was not an option.

The psychiatrist said to the service user, "How are you feeling?"

"Fine," was the reply.

Before the carers knew it, their son was discharged. This was not a good example of working together and discussing the finer details of a complex situation.

I was invited to give a presentation, to over twenty consultant psychiatrists, at an event that was led by one of the senior management team. The whole purpose of this talk was for me, as a carer, to highlight the need of professionals to work together with carers. One of the outcomes of this talk was an offer from several psychiatrists to come along and speak to our members of the Carers Action Group, which they did.

The Carers Action Group became the main consultation group for health professionals and management, and they came to our meetings when they wanted opinions, ideas and suggestions from carers on new policies, procedures, systems and planning. This was a massive and much-needed leap into professionals, carers and service users working together with the key aspect of looking at a service user's life holistically. Conveying the pertinent and meaningful reflections of the carers' lived experiences in induction videos for new staff was, and I believe still is, an invaluable part of public involvement and working together.

Through public involvement, I had the opportunity and the privilege, as a carer representative of the LCAG, to sit on many other boards and committees, in order to highlight the barriers carers experience. Meetings included discussions on inpatient safety, conferences on the Mental Health Act, clinical governance, recruitment and strategic planning groups, along with training and delivering the Positive Living and Understanding Schizophrenia (PLUS) course, in addition to writing articles pertaining to service user and carer involvement.

There is another aspect that I have not mentioned yet and that is the service of the Carer Development Support Team, established to help and support carers. I personally have to say that this was a brilliant initiative. Without this team and its support workers, carers would have had no one to talk to, or listen to us, in addition to their advice and guidance all those years ago. I always said, and still say now, that the care support workers that I have had over many years were, at that time, my saving grace.

When Leeds Mental Health started to apply for foundation trust status, I was one of the carer governors participating in the strategic planning. I, like many others, strongly believed that a more holistic approach needed to be discussed and acted upon when providing services for people with mental health difficulties. I kept hammering this home at practically every meeting I attended; to the point that they must have got fed up of hearing about it, but they never expressed that.

Through my own experiences as a carer, it was certainly one of the aspects of mental healthcare at that time which was so obviously missing. They were successful with their application for foundation trust status, and I have to give credit where credit is due, the CEO, Chris Butler, and all his staff, carers and service users involved worked incredibly hard. It really does give me great pleasure to say that I thoroughly enjoyed being part of that process, and although services for improvement were ongoing, due to the proactiveness of all, the services advanced immensely after this achievement.

**Campaigning:** in its different forms has been going on for decades and for all sorts of injustices, including politics, policies and laws in government, and other establishments, involving carers' rights, all of which understandably results in frustration and anger and the drive to put life right.

The issue of mental health has, over the last decade, become a subject we can talk about openly now, and the climate for recognition of needs has changed, however, has it changed enough? Various organisations campaign on behalf of carers' rights, one of them being Carers UK. They state: *'We have a long history and our past has firmly shaped how Carers UK operates today. We owe everything to the vision, commitment and values of the carers who led the organisation through its infancy'.*

Carers have a lot to thank Mary Webster for when she gave up working as a Congregational minister in 1954 (the year that I was born) to care for her parents, at just thirty-one years of age. She spent many years thinking about her situation and the disadvantages, not least financial, that it had created.

I was only nine years old when Mary Webster promptly addressed the public on her situation, the practical difficulties, the isolation and financial hardship that women carers were encountering, a situation for carers that was unexposed, and that an organisation was needed to address these issues. Mary formed the National Council for the Single Woman and her

Dependants in 1965 and, over the following few years, she demonstrated an acute political intuitiveness for selecting accurate allies. With the help of some key political professionals, the council won the first ever legislative change with the 1967 Dependent Relative Tax.

Sadly, Mary Webster died in 1969 at the age of forty-six. I was fifteen at the time and enjoying my teenage years with very little thought of the future. However, four years later, I was married, and five years later I had my second child and became a carer. It did not take me long to fully understand the significance of Mary Webster's clear-sighted and genius approach to the needs of carers.

In 2001, the Carers National Association was renamed Carers UK with Imelda Redmond CBE appointed as chief executive officer. Leeds was but one of the very many branches managed by Carers UK. This accomplished organisation, valuable in its work for carers, hold carers' conferences annually which gives all carers an opportunity to meet with many other carers from branches throughout the country.

Through my dear friend, David Proudlove (one of the most dedicated, loyal, humorous and admirable carers I have ever met) invited me on to the committee of the Carers UK Leeds Branch, and I had no hesitation in accepting. It was there that I, once again, had the opportunity to meet and get to know many more carers, all in diverse situations and circumstances but with the same aim, to improve and campaign for carers' rights.

David cares for his wife, Dee. They both have a wonderful sense of humour and have become cherished and dear friends. My husband and I applaud and commend them both in the way in which they both deal with life and its problems, yet they brush aside their own difficulties to ask about us and our son. Whatever life is throwing at us at the time, when we visit them Dee will make us laugh with her quick-witted and amusing humour.

I will never forget the way in which all the other members encouraged and supported me to fight one of the most harrowing and horrendous injustices I have had to face, when I was accused of being fraudulent in using online banking for my son. Not only did all the other members make me feel welcome, but they encouraged and supported me in my Better Banking Campaign for Carers.

From joining the Leeds branch, I attended the Carers UK conferences in London every year, if possible, and had the pleasure of meeting and working with Madeleine Starr, Director of Business, Development and Innovation, in various events. Former CEOs Imelda Redmond, Helena Herklots, chair, David Grayson and all staff at Carers UK were all extremely supportive. One lady in particular, who introduced herself to me at a conference, was Dame Philippa Russell, formerly the chair of the Prime Minister's Standing Commission on Carers, who again supported me with her constant communication and encouragement. Everyone I spoke to could not believe the injustice I was facing, yet they understood what I was going through and were willing to help.

Never in my wildest dreams could I have imagined that being a carer would take me on a journey into a world of radio interviews, television, parliament, speaking at conferences, hosting events and receiving awards, along with meeting so many lovely people. However, it is the carers of this world that have so much to deal with when looking after every aspect of a service user's life and, if you are facing an injustice right now, please remember that whatever we face in life as carers we can, and will, question and challenge all the unfairness thrown at us, we just have to face the oppositionist with as much commitment, care, attention, dedication and strength that we give our loved ones, and those are many powerful and almighty attributes, just used in a different set of circumstances.

*'Never underestimate your problem or your ability to deal with it.'* – Robert H. Schuller

## History of Carers UK Leeds Branch

Judy Fitton was very active in setting up the Carers Centre, which became Carers Leeds. Jean Townsend was its first manager and strongly supported Carers UK. In 1978, the national organisation was the National Council for the Single Woman and her Dependents, as mentioned earlier. In 1981 the chair, Miss Oldham, broadcast on Radio Leeds and in 1982 she was on ITV.

Mary Gilbourne then became the secretary who it is stated compiled a keeping house list of reliable workmen, this was an early forerunner of the Keeping House List. In 1985, the National Council had collaborated with the World of Property Housing Trust to set up two warden-assisted housing schemes, one of which was in Leeds – The Oakfield Housing Scheme. These are thought to have been some of the first sheltered housing schemes in the country. Leeds Branch was congratulated on its contribution to the successful outcome. [*Copyright Carers UK Leeds Branch Newsletter*]

**Carers Leeds** was established in 1996 and is an independent charity. Their expert and experienced staff give specialist and tailored support, along with advice and information, to unpaid carers aged over sixteen. An organisation that is outstanding in its work, unquestionably dedicated to improving the lives of thousands of carers in Leeds and led by an exceptional, down-to-earth, outstanding chief executive officer, Val Hewison, who strives to ensure that the services carers need, and much more, are in place. If you are a carer needing help and support contact Carers Leeds at advice@carersleeds.org.uk. At the time of writing this book, the total number of unpaid carers in Leeds is 72,000. In England, the total at the moment is 7 million, Northern Island is 213,980, Scotland's figure is 759,000 and Wales with 370,000 carers. These figures are increasing every day.

# CHAPTER 2

# What is a Social Injustice?

*'Never be afraid to raise your voice for honesty and truth and compassion against injustice and lying and greed.'* – William Faulkner

## Unfair, Problem, Complaint or Injustice

<u>Unfair:</u> a] Not based on or behaving according to the principles of equality and justice.

b] Not following the rules of a game or sport: 'he was sent off for unfair play'. [*Oxford Dictionaries Online*]

<u>Problem:</u> A matter or situation regarded as unwelcome or harmful and needing to be dealt with and overcome. [*Oxford Dictionaries Online*]

<u>Complaint:</u> Any expression of dissatisfaction, whether oral or written, and whether justified or not. [*FCA*]

<u>Injustice:</u>

Practical Injustice: relating to unfairness or undeserved outcomes, the term may be applied in reference to a particular event or situation. [*Wikipedia*]

Moral and Social Injustice: based on a system of personal values and beliefs rather than legal punishments and retributions closely related to Social Injustice. [*Google*]

Change or a lack of change in policies, systems, procedures and laws are constant barriers to carers, despite numerous pieces of information in leaflets, booklets and websites covering a wide range of issues from benefits and care support, to funding in care homes, we would expect to find something from this information that carers can use constructively.

From my experience, this is not always the case, as there are too many small and scattered pockets of information which do not give us the bigger picture of what we need to know, and invariably there will be some information missing which then requires us to find more.

Joined-up thinking, between organisations and the government, is required in order to produce a more comprehensive structure on services when we are dealing with the many aspects of our loved one's lives. It is these complexities, and the emotions that go with manoeuvring around and tackling a social injustice, that I want to raise and question so that in future we can take these unnecessary, distressing and stressful experiences and turn them into positive ones.

In the mid 1950s, I was frequently on the receiving end of the teacher's cane for forgetting my times tables, along with being punished for being left-handed. This punishment was given by way of a cane being brandished over one's knuckles pretty hard. Is this kind of punishment an injustice or unfair? Whatever you think, it would certainly never be considered now. I believe discipline has its place in society, but the effect it had on me for being a 'cack-hander', as left-handers were called in those days, was the feeling of being the odd kid out. At primary and junior school, I remember trying to hold back the tears, as the cane met the sensitive flesh of my small hand just because I wrote left-handed, but as soon as I got home and told my mum, the tears would flow. The stigma of being left-handed was continued in secondary school. However, my English and drama teachers were the best a child could wish for. They knew how to be firm but kind, to laugh with us and to stimulate our imaginations; all in all, two outstanding educators. I loved those subjects, and I did not need any motivation in writing plays and essays of fifteen or more pages.

People do come face to face with numerous injustices in connection with corporate businesses, health and social care, and independent business. For example, finances, support agencies, care homes, general practitioners, pharmacists, hospitals, and many more, often instigated by people with surly attitudes, a lack of understanding and intolerance, along with policies and systems that are not designed to recognise carers when acting on behalf of their loved ones. Have you ever been faced with an injustice?

Carers can be forgiven when they let an injustice they are confronted with pass by. They are too tired to deal with it, too exhausted to debate the facts of the injustice, too stressed to fight their corner and, unfortunately, some organisations prey on this vulnerability knowing that if they wait long enough the carer will not carry the complaint through, but if you do, they may offer you a couple of hundred pounds straight away to get rid of the complaint.

In order to achieve results, we have to be resilient and persistent. Just like our loved ones, we too need stability, commitment, competence, understanding, compassion and care in order to have peace of mind and live with the reassuring knowledge that we can depend on others to do their job efficiently and effectively.

Carers' experiences come from a variety of different perspectives, regardless of whether or not they have a legal duty to manage finances. Problems and issues, large or small, we have the choice to either question, challenge, complain, or simply do nothing at all. But I ask, as many carers do, why do we have to fight for common sense and logic in the first place?

Conceivably, by exploration and innovation on all these aspects, we can as carers highlight our practical concerns and issues. When we know we are right, we stand a good chance of getting the injustice resolved. We also rely on the recipient of the complaint to demonstrate excellent moral and social values, as well as their expertise in the organisation they work for, to address and make good our issues. Many barriers can be eliminated by organisations reviewing their existing services and products with the carer in mind.

I have helped carers and service users, on many occasions, who struggle with part, or all, of this procedure to write letters of complaint, which is why I have included hints and tips in this chapter on writing a complaint, in the hope that it will help, in some small way, if you ever have to write your first one, without it seeming too daunting a task.

## What Can I Do When Faced with a Social Injustice?

## Hints and Tips

Carers have to deal with a multitude of issues. If you find yourself dealing with an injustice, the following format may help in getting organised with just where you need to start to deal with a problem. Whatever injustice you are facing in your caring situation, however small or large, writing the problem down in a logical order will give you a clearer picture; this in turn will give you the confidence to articulate your issue/s to those concerned.

## How Will That Help Me?

Written evidence is vital in dealing with injustices and, with all the facts of your complaint in front of you, which can include your own personal feelings and the effect this problem has had on you, in addition to other relevant information, you are building up your chain of reasoning which supports your side of the situation, thereby being able to present your case with a coherent and logical approach. This format will promote confidence in presenting a complaint because, having it all written down, you can be sure and safe in the knowledge that you are not going to forget one little detail.

An injustice can make us feel that an organisation is covering something up, important information that we are not being given, and the result of this is that, as carers, we are left feeling disillusioned, powerless, hurt, isolated, confused, weary, angry, cautious and distrusting. Yet we have to stay calm, hopeful, optimistic, persistent and assertive, in order to find the strength to fight for justice for our loved ones.

**Hints and Tips on Making a Formal Complaint**

Get Your Facts Right

When you make a formal complaint, follow the company's complaints procedure and see it through to a final conclusion. If you find this is difficult to do on your own, seek help from a relevant organisation that can help you with advice and support.

**How Do I Start?**

Well, I know this is pretty obvious, but you will need a folder/ file, notebook and pen. Relevant notes need to be kept, hence the notebook, as does all relevant documentation which you can save in your case file. Keep everything in one place, so you know exactly where it is when you need it. Safeguarding all correspondence relating to a complaint that you send to a company and vice versa is essential.

Many times, over the years, I have been dealing with several complaints at once which meant I had several case files, consisting of two and three folders, all named with the title of the complaint and the company I was dealing with. I know when my paperwork is organised, I feel organised mentally.

Approach the construction of your complaint in a logical order

**Covering Letter:** Introductory covering letter in which you can state the relevant details of the names and addresses of the person/s involved along with the title of the incident. Conclude your covering letter by saying that you are enclosing a full statement of events, along with the issues arising from them that you wish to be addressed, and that you trust your formal complaint will be taken seriously.

- **Beginning of report:** Give a full explanation of the nature of your complaint including the events leading up to the main incident. Include any relevant conversations, comments, or remarks that were made at the time, in addition to dates, times and places.

- **Middle:** Identify and write down all the main issues of your complaint that have arisen from it. Underneath each of the issues write 'Action:' and explain, briefly and concisely, exactly how you would like to see the issues addressed, for example this may be a written apology, or an action that needs to be taken on something in order to rectify the problem.

- **Conclusion:** This is the final part of your report in which again you can reiterate that you trust your official complaint will be investigated thoroughly and that you look forward to hearing from them/or '*I await your reply*'. End with '*Yours sincerely*' if you have used a person's name or '*Yours faithfully*' if you have used '*Dear Sir/Madam*'. Check grammar and spellings; it all adds to the professionalism of your report.

Useful reminders to put in your notebook:

- Research the issue you are complaining about if you feel it is necessary for your complaint.
- Ensure all facts are true, correct and in order.
- Think about what help and support/action you need to assist you in making your complaint, if any.
- Seek advice from a professional, if you need to, before you start. You have the right to have an advocate with you, if you wish, if you attend a meeting.
- When writing your complaint, stick to the main issues and principles of it, don't get bogged down or sidetracked by irrelevant conversations.
- Be absolutely certain of the main point of your complaint.
- Write down your experience, as soon as possible, whilst the facts are fresh in your mind.
- What happened?
- When did it happen?
- How did it happen?
- Why did it happen?
- Write down all your issues and concerns.
- The sequence of your covering letter.
- The sequence of your report.
- Use a logical order.
- Write down dates, times, names, addresses and contact numbers.
- Write down roles and responsibilities of the person you are dealing with. If you do not think they are the right person to deal with your concerns, talk to a more senior person.
- Keep a record of all telephone conversations, with whom you spoke, what they said, along with the time and date the call was made.
- Ensure you ask for everything in writing from the person

you are making the complaint to whether it is by email or letter.

- Write down the impact your experience has had/is having on you and/or the person you care for/family/friends.
- Write down what action you would like to see taken in order to resolve the complaint.
- Check the 'Carers Rights' policy along with any other policies and procedures that relate to your complaint. If you are not sure about this, contact the appropriate professional to help you.
- If necessary for your complaint, speak to your local authority Adult Health and Social Care Services.
- You can include statements such as: *'I would be interested to know what suggestions and actions your company can sanction in terms of resolving these issues in the interest of both parties.'*
- Obtain all the relevant facts. if needed, in connection with the company's customer service policy in order to ascertain what particular clause your complaint refers to.
- Request a meeting.

If the company you are dealing with invites you to a meeting to discuss the complaint further and you decide to go, you do have the right to take an advocate with you, if you wish. Having got this far with a complaint, it is my experience that a face-to-face meeting will accomplish the penultimate stage of a complaint, when the final agreements on any action can be decided and put into place there and then, or at least as soon as possible, depending on the nature of your concerns.

I have always attended these kinds of meetings, and on occasions I have been the one to instigate them. As a rule, I have found them to be very proactive and constructive in moving the matter forward, often bringing about a final conclusion in terms of an answer, action, settlement and/or reimbursement, or an action which is appropriate to the benefit of both parties.

In order to help anyone, organisations should strive to achieve and commit to excellence and good practice, and this means working together, listening and addressing issues, giving accurate information, support and advice, in addition to being proactive in demonstrating genuine understanding and compassion in order to achieve a satisfactory outcome.

Face-to-face meetings also have the advantage of being introduced and speaking to the people you are dealing with and, more often than not, it is normally at this stage that it will be senior management.

One of the benefits of a meeting is that it is not as time-consuming as continually writing letters, and given the fact that you have got this far with your complaint, because most of it will have been discussed by phone, letter, email, etc. anyway, all parties know exactly where the starting point will be when you arrive for it.

Everyone present should be made to feel welcome and at ease, along with being given the opportunity to ask additional questions, make comments and clarify issues if you are not clear about them. It is a good idea to make a list of these other questions before the meeting and take it with you so you don't forget them, and I do not say this in any critical way of one's memory, it is because, if you are like me, your stomach will already have that many butterflies, not fluttering around but thrashing around, which sends my nerves into overdrive, that deep breaths are in order here, and you might be entitled to forget an odd question. The meeting should be a civilised, amicable and democratic one, which in turn produces results.

If you remain dissatisfied that the complaint has not been completely resolved, then I would expect the company to inform you of what the next step would be. They may have other suggestions towards a solution, if not, it maybe that you yourself will have to write to the ombudsman, or obtain further help and support from your local or regional advice centres. Whatever you do, be confident, proactive and persistent, and don't give up.

Research suggests that the common cause of injustice is human selfishness. Exploring the reasons behind this, I ponder whether this is because some people do not take their role seriously at work and dodge what could be a time-consuming query, an event just to acknowledge a person sometimes seems too much for some people, let alone any perception of what people go through in their lives. Could it be that they are just not interested in other people's issues at all? If this is the case, human selfishness eliminates any hopes of the recipient being listened to and treated with respect. I have been on the receiving end of such selfishness on many occasions, however, on the positive, productive and meaningful side of the fence, I have had the pleasure of seeking help from people and professionals who are non-judgemental, open-minded and kind-hearted, who go that 'extra mile' to resolve an issue.

Please note this is a fictional case

**Example Covering Letter**

---

Private and Confidential

*Sender's name and address*

*Recipient's name and address*

For the attention of:

Date

Re: *Title of your complaint*

Formal Letter of complaint in connection with an incident on the 21.12.2019 due to dietary requirements being disregarded for Edwin Stewart, 46 Banner Street, Whistdown, ES28 OHNO.

Dear [Name of the person you are writing to. If you do not have a particular name then address your letter to the senior manager/manager],

**Beginning/Introduction:** This is your opening paragraph. Start by introducing yourself and that you are writing in connection with an incident/issue which took place/happened at [state place/venue].

**Middle:** This is the main issue of your complaint, stick to all the facts at this point and include names, dates and times. What happened and who was involved.

**Issues Arising:** Bullet point all the issues arising from your complaint that you would like addressing e.g. the way that [insert name if you have one] a member of staff dealt with my enquiry was surly and abrupt instead of being professional and helpful...

You may find you have only one or two issues to be addressed or there may be ten or twenty. As you list them, number them if you have quite a few, as this helps for future reference when discussing in a meeting or verbally over the phone.

**Resolution:** There may be specific resolutions that you want to see to each one of the issues you have raised, so you will need to add what action you believe should be taken to address them. There may be other issues that you would like advice on, so you could also add those if needed. E.g. I would be most grateful if you could inform me of what suggestions your organisation has in terms of resolving these issues in the interest of both parties concerned.

**Final Paragraph:** I trust that this, my official letter of complaint, will be given serious consideration, and I look forward to hearing from you as promptly as possible.

**Yours sincerely,**

**Case Scenario**
Discuss this scenario and the issues it raises. What can be done to resolve this complaint to the benefit of all parties? Use this scenario to devise a complaint letter using the template letter provided and the hints and tips.

**Background**: Edwin, aged thirty-four, attends a day centre for adults with severe learning difficulties. In this case, Edwin has been given a sugary drink by staff at lunchtime despite what it says on his care plan. However, Edwin attended his dance and drama session straight after lunch. He thoroughly enjoys this activity, has a vivid imagination, works well with his peers and contributes to the group activity in a positive way despite his limitations.

The dance session started with an improvisation of movements to 'Ghostbusters', in which Edwin was running and dashing around and demonstrating impulsive behaviour. The session ended with slower movements to 'Lion King'. However, Edwin insisted on being the lion, and consequently ran around the room roaring and growling loudly, scaring the other four students.

In a short scene from *Romeo and Juliet*, Edwin's imagination ran riot and he insisted he be Romeo. He stood behind a chair, his makeshift balcony, pretending to look down from it, towards Juliet who was played by Catherine.

He stretched his arm downwards and towards her, his hand reaching out to take hers, at the same time as bellowing out, "Romeo, Romeo wherefore art thou..." Whereupon, Catherine, rebuffing his gesture, wandered to the other side of the room, a bit put out, because it should have been her saying the lines.

Edwin moved from behind the chair, and he then proceeded to take off his clothes. For his safety and dignity, the staff quickly and calmly restored order. The manager informed Edwin's mother, Mary, and Edwin's carer of thirty-four years, that due to his behaviour he should be excluded from the centre for the next two weeks.

Mary told the manger that she was not happy about this decision and wondered what had prompted Edwin's behaviour to be so extreme. He had problems like all the other students, but they had always been dealt with in a proper manner, as all the staff were trained to teach severe learning difficulty students.

Mary asked what Edwin had had for lunch for that day, and when she discovered that he had had a very sugary drink, complained that he should never have been given this. It clearly stated on his care plan that he was not allowed this kind of beverage, as it resulted in exactly the type of behaviour they said he was displaying, so to exclude Edwin from the class he loved participating in, to which, up until now, he had never been any trouble, was clearly the fault of someone ignoring a care plan in terms of his dietary requirements.

After an investigation, it transpired that the care worker on duty that day was a new member of staff and had never been advised of this dietary requirement for Edwin, at the same time, this new member of staff, also fully trained in teaching special needs students, never bothered to look at the care plan.

As we are aware, too much sugar is not good for us and in Edwin's case, due to underlying health problems, food or drink high in refined sugar exacerbated his hyperactivity and aggressive behaviour. This is because sugars and carbohydrates enter the bloodstream quickly, causing rapid changes in blood sugar levels, which may make a person more active. Research has been carried out in this particular area by various professionals but have contrasting opinions.

**One of my formal complaints from a Lived Experience**

At the time of starting the complaint, my parents were in different hospitals and, on discharge, moved to different care homes. My complaint was still ongoing and took three years to resolve.

From day one, the organisations involved with my father's care, there followed an extensive catalogue of errors. Our formal complaint exceeded approximately fifty plus pages. It was an exceptionally challenging, distressing and immensely frustrating time in which we highlighted forty-six issues.

I informed the organisations that I was going to make a formal complaint; I received a consent form which had to be signed by my father before the complaint could be dealt with.

I strongly object to these kind of consent forms, because a] on the one hand it has been said that my father cannot make decisions due to his severe Alzheimer's, and on other occasions like this it is said he has the capacity to sign a consent form. And b] it is me who is making the complaint about the competence and inefficiency of the department and its provision, which my father would be oblivious to, therefore this is an unfathomable and contradictory consent form, and I cannot help but feel that, in certain circumstances, rules are reshaped to suit a particular set of needs. I explained to Dad what this form was for and he signed it, however, retention of Dad's memory was, in layman's terms, nanoseconds. I duly sent the consent form back, making my disapproval known. Consequently, my novel of official complaints followed in February 2014, to which I then receive a letter stating that all the issues I had raised would be investigated.

These are just a few of the complaints on that list:
- Home visits and professional conduct within a patient's home
- Home visits by community psychiatric nurse (CPN)
- Care plans
- Outpatient appointments
- Appointment letters
- Capacity report
- Social services
- Advocacy
- Care review meeting
- Minutes of meetings
- Medical records
- Leadership and meetings
- Communication with patient
- Continuity

There were several issues for each one of the complaints put forward and, as I said, the list was not exhaustive by any means. It became apparent very quickly that a lack of leadership, mixed messages, verbal and written communication with errors, along with inappropriate attitudes, and a lack of professionalism in all aspects of this complaint were present. The professional investigating this complaint was proactive and efficient.

So what happened? We received fifteen apologies in response to the first letter of complaint and seventeen apologies in response to the second letter of the complaint. The number of records and information which had not been kept, recorded or updated totalled an unbelievable nineteen instances. Out of thirty-seven apologies given, the family accepted seven and the rest were acknowledged, but not accepted.

Further responses from the organisation were not satisfactory, thereby instigating a second investigation. My reply referred, amongst other things, to unsatisfactory answers to some of the questions and queries we'd put to them, along with outlining the issues that seemed to have just been ignored totally. Their replies, for one reason or another, some of them acceptable, took time to materialise. After a lengthy period of a sequence of letters being sent and responses coming back, because of staff moving, leaving, or retiring in between, we were getting nowhere. I sent the following letter to the organisation which briefly summed up the last several years of correspondence and investigations.

*Further to your letter dated ..., I forward to you my response. I strongly believe that, yet again, none of the issues I have raised through this extremely stressful and lengthy period have been addressed properly.*

*In both responses, Mr ... has investigated, reviewed, revised, recognised and acknowledged. They have accepted and apologised, all of which are futile, not practical, or based on the situation as it really is. Therefore ... and I would like a meeting to discuss these issues further.*

In response to this letter, a meeting was arranged. With a degree of apprehension, we met with a multidisciplinary team and management who were amicable and welcoming. Round the table action points were addressed and fulfilled.

After a couple of hours, we walked out of the building into the sunshine and breathed a sigh of relief, knowing that our time in all this and the valid points we raised on forty-six accounts had not been in vain. The organisation stated that they had learned lessons from this lengthy dispute, which they would use to improve communication and provision, as well as involving carers more.

If you have been in the right all along justice will prevail, not only will you have accomplished what you set out to do, but you may even have helped change the way systems, policies and procedures work for the better, not just for your loved one but for other vulnerable people and their carers too.

# CHAPTER 3

# Do I Look Invisible?

*'Ignore me, I don't care. I'm used to it anyways. I am invisible.'* – Unknown [*Pinterest*]

Look into the eyes of a carer, and there you will see the tiredness and the hopelessness of a situation that no one seems to want to know about, or that no one can help us with our hidden fears, angst and unease that is sometimes at the forefront of our mind, or a little bit deeper down, depending on how the day is going. Yet on the other hand, when a person does genuinely help with an issue, they must surely see the realisation and recognition on the carer's face, that this person truly wants to help, and the relief that their support gives them.

Excluding the professionals who work with carers, I focus mainly on the bigger, outside world, when I ask the question, do I look invisible?

Yes, I do, because very often I feel like a faceless and indiscernible entity. I have felt like this many times, especially when speaking with people who have no concept of what a carer's life entails, so they change the subject or start talking about themselves, to detract from the sensitive, distressing and humbling nature of my dialogue. My knowledge and involvement of the realities of life, exposes their own insensitivity, incomprehension and sometimes intolerance, simply because the nature of a carer's life is uncomfortable for them to listen to.

It can also be a relentless fight with non-carers and professionals, whom a carer has to deal with on behalf of the service user. It is not very often we talk about what happens practically, physically or emotionally behind the scenes in our lives, in just the same way as others do not always detect the fear, worry and apprehension if we do.

We may sometimes tell others snippets of our experiences, even revealing a bit more of it to a trusted friend, and this can be positive and helpful.

Some people do not think about what they are going to say before they say it, they do not stop to think about whether what they are about to say is appropriate and helpful, and if it isn't the consequences can cause a lot of hurt.

Many of the lived experiences I write about leave me saying "It beggars belief", when I am left feeling appalled at some of the statements that have been made to me.

When discussing issues with some people, their body language gives us a great deal of information, and when they try to have a dialogue about carers' issues, it soon becomes apparent that they are not knowledgeable enough to discuss any of them, and then they try to defend their inappropriate words and actions, leaving the carer feeling incredibly frustrated and angry; the sheer lack of seeing carers, for who we are and what we do, ultimately makes us feel invisible and inconsequential.

Well here's a revelation for those who see carers in this light, thinking that we only have tales of woe to convey; we are human beings, individuals who have skills and qualities, just like anyone else. We are people who have achieved something in our lives, be it devoting a life of caring for our loved ones and/or something unique and personal we have achieved for ourselves. Yet very often, our faces and persona are unseen by people who do not even try to understand or worse do not want to know.

However, I say, with dedication and conviction, that caring has immense rewards in terms of being able to help someone less fortunate than oneself, in terms of sharing laughter, problems, tears and achievements with my loved one.

Even though a carer's role is acknowledged much more in society these days by various, professional carer organisations who play a vital role in the well-being of carers, by having drop-in centres, one-to-one sessions, or in outreach work, these are the people who positively, and beyond any shadow of a doubt, understand carers. They do not underestimate the role of the carer, so I reckon it goes without saying that we are much more at ease in knowing these people are friends and are here to help and support when we need them.

**I care. Do you?**

*Most of the time I sort the queries and paperwork out,*
*Myself, at home*
*On my own, alone*
*Sometimes I need to see an expert to help me complete the*
*task*
*That's all I ask*
*I do this for my loved one, who does not understand*
*So all I need is a helping hand*
*This is the problem I explain*
*Will my venture be in vain?*
*You sit with hand on chin and ponder for a while*
*There is no acknowledgement, or smile*
*Hmm, you say, you act on this person's behalf, do you have*
*proof?*
*He said this so aloof*
*I took the document out of my bag*
*Here we go, I thought as my hopes began to sag*
*He raised his head; our records do not state that you are a*
*carer*
*And caring*
*But this proves I am, and I'm sharing*
*This evidence with you*
*Our systems and procedures don't allow us to do what you*
*ask*
*Why, what is so hard about this, your technology cannot*
*grasp?*
*We went around in a loop dialogue*
*Getting nowhere, wading through smog*
*Over an hour of him saying no and me saying yes*
*Why is this issue so hard to address?*

*My heart is quickly beating, my pulse racing*
*Frustration and anger pacing*
*If I speak up please do not see this as a confrontation*
*I just need your help in this situation*
*He stands up*
*An action that tells me he has had enough*
*Yet another barrier*
*Yet another rebuff*
*I walk away with a lump in my throat*
*It's raining now and I haven't got a coat*
*Yet again I have been made to feel different*
*Isolated and out of line*
*A leftover*
*A nonentity from the history of time*
*Please don't try to tell me what you think I need*
*I am an intelligent person, not a dead weed*
*I know something can be done about this situation*
*All it needs is your care and cooperation*
*I can only hope that sometime soon*
*People strive to help*
*And then I'll be over the moon*

*I Care. Do You?*

# CHAPTER 4

# A Carer's Analogy

Trying to make any sense of life as we care, especially when dealing with other problems, never really gives us time to sit and think. When I did have a little time to write, I decided to write my own analogy which, for me, was very therapeutic.

**I am a Carer. My life is like a River.**

'*Have you also learned that secret from the river; that there is no such thing as time? That the river is everywhere at the same time, at the source and at the mouth, at the waterfall, at the ferry, at the current, in the ocean and in the mountains...*' – Hermann Hesse

I am soothed, by the serenity of beauty all around me, huge, green slopes reaching for the sky with no hidden, rough rocks, relaxing into a moment of calmness. Washing away the tiredness, with the intermittent and most welcome wisps of cool breezes, yet letting the warmth of the sun soothe me.

Lying down on the worn-out piece of banking that houses a patch of warm, light sand, I stare in wonder at the glazed pebbles shining like silk, as the gentle ripple of water burbles at the river's edge. Dozing, I listen to the sounds of the countryside, as the water trickles over my toes. Let me listen and sleep to the placid and hypnotic sounds of Mother Nature. Then another unexpected predicament occurs.

The river is never still, always on the move, always changing, taking me with it on its journey. Forever unpredictable, never complacent, as the waters gurgle and deepen. Fast-flowing and diverting along its way, a journey of uncertainty. Shocking, frightening, when suddenly the river snakes into a magnificent expanse of openness, a vast mirror capturing every reflection.

All seems calm, as the water glides silently, picking up pace on its journey. Some of the fallen trees I can clear, and even dodge the low branches, but many others trap me, catch me, slow me down and, at times, even stop me, but not for long.

River rising, swirling, around a bend a series of rapids, nothing serious I hope but all too easy to drop one's guard, and when you do, you end up pointing in the wrong direction and fighting to get back into the mainstream section.

Twisting, whirling, skies misting, playing out its own drama as it swells with pride, trembling as it competes with the rapids and waterfalls, roaring and crashing. Advancing towards the consequences of this turmoil now seems insurmountable. Stopper waves, where massive strength is needed to escape. Frustrated, cold and upset, a situation I have not been in before and never want to experience again. I tell myself I am not scared of any impending whirlpools which can now suck me under so that I lose my breath.

Just for a few moments, peace and quiet, until I hear the stupendous and thunderous sound from the waterfalls. A brook tumbling, a rapid crashing, the little stream burbling, gentle raindrops, and mountainous snow are melting. The river nears the sea, divided into a delta with hundreds of different channels. Are they all navigable? Which do I take? Just what is the best course of action?

**What is your Carer's Analogy?**

# CHAPTER 5

# Carers' Qualities and Skills

*"How do you like your fried eggs, Mum?" "Boiled please."*

Demonstrating patience at the end of the day is no soiree when looking after Mum. I help her sit down on the chair at the dinner table and, as always, she needs to be further up to the table, or she will end up with more dinner in her lap than in her mouth.

"I'm going to move you a bit further up, Mum, so you will have to help me by lifting your bottom up a little from the chair, because it is too heavy to move both you and the chair at the same time."

Mum does not lift her bum up from the chair but proceeds to move only the top half of her body, in a forward rocking motion, to give the appearance that she is advancing towards the table, at the same time making a profound, very deep grunt, snort, huffing and puffing sound, as she strives to put every ounce of energy into the movement when in fact she is not budging an inch. I now get the impression that I am trying to coax a stubborn pig from its mud bath, not my mum to the table for dinner.

*Employ your wonderful sense of humour*, says my inner voice. So I do.

When I finally get Mum in the correct position to eat, I say, "Right, Mum, would you like a trough or a plate?" We all burst out laughing.

Our sense of humour is vital at any time but none more so than when we are caring. What could potentially be an exasperating and quarrelsome scene, laughter can suddenly defuse.

Let us bear in mind that carers do not apply for an unpaid carer's role. There is no hard copy of a job description, because we know what needs doing and when we have to do it. We do not have a recognised CV for this role, or indeed appropriate qualifications or degree. In addition to our timetable, we have to be prepared for the unexpected turn of events which may occur on a regular basis. Yet we have excellent qualifications and résumés, along with many other attributes, such as aptitude, expertise, skills and knowledge on our specialist subject.

Furthermore, we do not have a union we can go to for advice and guidance, or to help us with all the general and formal issues and complexities that caring brings when there is an injustice. I have, on many occasions, stated to the boards and committees I am on that we need an independent governing body that supports carers, just like employment needs a workers' union.

Carers are people, individuals, who have their own likes, dislikes, hobbies, work, families and so on, just like anybody else. Yet many of us have been in situations trying to resolve problems, asking questions, explaining predicaments, with responses that are patronising and makes one feel like an idiot.

Over the forty plus years I have been caring, I have had the privilege of meeting hundreds of carers, and instantaneously there is already an exclusive affinity, because we already have the fundamentals of our role in common, that massive chunk of commonality pertaining to each and every area of caring, a mutual understanding of the human emotions we encounter as a result of our lived experiences.

I strongly believe that our qualities and skills should be showcased and in this chapter I do just that, in the hope that we will be treated by others for who we are as individuals and as carers, with qualities and skills that must never be undermined or lost, because our individuality is paramount to our well-being; it is who we are.

Many carers have made me laugh when relaying their own caring experiences. In the same way, their deeply moving stories bring tears to my eyes. I sincerely empathise with my fellow carers at the crises they are going through, the injustices they are dealing with, yet still my fellow carer smiles despite the stress and tiredness they feel, but would go to the core of the galaxy to get their loved one a Milky Way if that is what she/he has requested.

The following carers' lived experiences have been written or told by the carers themselves, along with their consent to be used in the publishing of this book.

**Written by Ann Petty – Carer**

*My husband and I were childhood sweethearts.*

My husband was diagnosed with Parkinson's disease several years ago, although I had noticed some signs of concern on odd days before that. (Situations may have changed since going into print.)

Prior to retirement, my husband was a senior quantity surveyor in private practice and, at times, this was a pressurised role with a high volume of work and constant deadlines to meet. I believe this took its toll on the last few years of his working life.

He is unlucky in that he has both the physical limitations of Parkinson's and also Parkinson's dementia. I am aware that symptoms vary widely, and each person is completely different in their response to the disease. In my husband's case, he experiences extreme fatigue every day, resulting in fluctuating difficulty in concentration and communication. I have noticed his dexterity is impaired and the daily newspaper can be a challenge. He now finds eating and using cutlery difficult, so I usually cut up food for him and avoid crispy bread.

Eating in company is stressful for him, as he is embarrassed about these difficulties, including excess saliva which gathers in his mouth and he is fearful of dribbling in public. His voice has become quieter, and he does have some swallowing difficulties at times.

He can be unsteady on his feet, and I worry constantly that he may fall, with the concern that a fall may produce further health problems. He uses a walking pole and has a 'stroller' for longer distances and outings. He does not appear to have a very marked 'tremor', but it becomes more obvious when he is tired. His body jerks frequently, and he requires some assistance with personal care and dressing.

From his point of view, the most distressing condition is in his mental decline, as he has always had a keen intellect and enquiring mind. This has been slowly impaired by his short-term memory loss and confusion, as he is no longer able to follow an instruction and retain recent conversation. He finds this extremely frustrating and upsetting, and I know this has been a source of great sadness to him. His long-term memory is largely intact, and he can remember facts and incidents throughout our relationship that I had long forgotten. He finds social situations very stressful, and he is unable to follow and keep up with conversation, often retreating within himself on these occasions.

Despite all these difficulties for us both, as his carer, I think I largely cope, though I cannot say there are not very difficult and stressful days. With this in mind, I try to make all appointments for the late morning or afternoon and take advantage of the electronic system for repeat prescriptions and home delivery from the pharmacist.

Much of our communication, as a couple, is non-verbal, and my just being there is very important to my husband. I try to be a good listener, treating him with a gentle and unthreatening approach, though accept I do not get this right every time. At these times, I rely on my mantra 'tomorrow is another day'.

Being a carer is an isolating role, and I have often experienced a sense of loneliness. I have also experienced a sense of loss, not just on my husband's behalf, but also my own sense of anticipatory grief for the future and a grief for how things were before. I worry, at times, about the affect this role is having on my own health and well-being.

We have wonderful support from our son and daughter, along with our daughter and son-in-law. I feel blessed that they both have insight, sensitivity and sound sense when offering support and guidance.

I believe strongly that it is important to engage with as much support from statutory and charity organisations, like the Parkinson Society www.parkinsons.org.uk and the brain injury association Headway www.headway.org.uk, as they have a wealth of help and understanding. The anecdotal suggestions and views from other people in similar circumstances can be invaluable. My husband and I were childhood sweethearts and have known each other for 55 years. It is my intention to care for him as long as he needs me, because I love him.

---

**Brian Boffey – Carer**

**He invented the Jelly Tot – How cool is that!**

Google Dr Brian Boffey, and you will find umpteen articles on Brian's career and achievements and it is well worth reading. Straight out of university, Professor Lawrence set Brian up with one of the best jobs he could have ever envisaged. York-based confectionary giants, Rowntree's contacted Professor Lawrence at the University of Sheffield to see if they had any specialists in the chemistry departments at that time. The professor put Brian forward and he got the job, going on to become one of the highest paid research scientists in the company at that time.

During his time with Rowntree's, at the age of 28, he inadvertently invented the humble Jelly Tot, trying to develop a way to produce a powdered jelly that set instantly when it was added to cold water, however, after much experimentation, he deemed the research to be a failure. The consequences of the experiment were tiny droplets, which he, initially, considered to be collateral damage. After flavour and colour were added to the droplets, within weeks, they were being sold across the country. Despite his Jelly Tot invention, Brian never pocketed a penny. He said in an interview with the *Yorkshire Evening Post* that: "*Rowntree's were very good to me, and I certainly do not mind not having been recognised as the man who invented Jelly Tots.*"

Carers UK Leeds Branch, David Proudlove, a carer himself, was the chair of this branch and is a very dear and long-standing friend of Brian's, both gentlemen very highly respected in the caring community.

I was delighted when David asked me to be on the committee of the Carers UK Leeds Branch, which I accepted, and in doing so I had the privilege of meeting Brian. He told me his story, and when I told him about this book I wanted to write, he gave me permission to include this article.

However, there is another side to Brian who is a carer and, on deciding that he was not going to take it easy in his retirement in 1986, he went on to dedicate his time to caring for others by driving thousands upon thousands of miles as a voluntary ambulance driver. This entailed pushing wheelchairs up mountains and fulfilling a ninety-three-year-old woman's last request to go to the East Coast, so she could dip her feet in the sea on Scarborough beach. His total dedication to helping others has seen him awarded the prestigious Leeds NHS Trust Volunteer of the Year Award in 2011 and Good Citizen Award by Horsforth Town Council in 2012.

A father of three grown-up children and one grandchild, the University of Sheffield will always have an extra-special place in his heart, as it was there he met his wife. Brian said, "I met Sylvia on a night out at the students unions. A coach full of nurses would be dropped off outside the union and Sylvia caught my eye." Sylvia's father, Edwin Barron, was the former head of botany in Sheffield and received an MSC Honorary Degree from the University of Sheffield in 1982.

---

### Kauser Iqbal – Carer

*I gave up my work as a nursery officer to care for my brothers and have been a full-time carer for twenty-two years to date.*

I care for my two disabled, adult brothers who both have the same disabilities. Namely these are microcephaly, epilepsy and challenging behaviour. Microcephaly is a medical condition in which the brain does not develop properly resulting in a shorter-than-normal head. This may result in intellectual disability along with poor motor and speech function. Epilepsy causes seizures. These seizures are bursts of electrical activity in the brain that temporarily affect how it works.

The Challenging Behaviour Foundation behaviour.org.uk Challenging behaviour is how we describe a range of behaviours which some people with severe learning disabilities may display to get their needs met. Some of these behaviours are eating inedible objects, such as pen tops and bedding. Destructive behaviours include self-injury, whilst hurting others can be hair pulling and hitting. Other behaviours demonstrated are spitting, rocking and running away.

At twelve years old, I became a carer for my two disabled brothers, and had three siblings under eight years of age, one of them being my sister. My main role was to entertain them. I remember vividly one of the early days of taking them out, with two of my siblings clinging on to my coat and the third one in a buggy. Alone with my thoughts, as I walked down a busy Dewsbury Road, I felt so scared and isolated. What I really wanted to do was play with my friend on her bike, or go to the library. Everywhere I went, my siblings came with me. I even sat my brother on a high wall, whilst I grabbed a couple of precious minutes to play with my friends. When I look back at what the consequences could have been, by popping my brother on top of the wall, they never entered my head, he could so easily have fallen off and hurt himself badly.

Years later, I was so happy when my parents arranged my marriage, at last no more caring, or so I thought. My brother moved to a residential home, but he was so unhappy there. My husband and I could not bear to see him so sad, could not bear to see him so downhearted, a sense of despair on his face that said I feel no hope. We brought him back to our home to live with us. Six months later, my other brother moved in with us too, and they were reunited again.

I knew that life would not be easy from this point on, just as it was when I was a little girl, however, I planned how I would care for my brothers, but what I did not anticipate was the lack of support and the demands my family would make on my everyday life. It got to the point where I felt I was in a big black hole.

On hearing about Carers Leeds, I decided to go and see them for support, and this resulted in my embarking on a six-week well-being course. I learnt about vital life skills and self-help resources which all empowered me to be where I am today. Carers Leeds is like my extended family who loves me for who I am, treating me with respect and dignity.

---

Kauser was a volunteer for over six years in the community, helping people from all multicultural and diverse communities, in order to help people achieve a better quality of life through health groups and training. She went on to develop Beeston Action for Families which is a service user and carer-led community group. As a coordinator for this group, Kauser helped to develop a DVD called *Loud and Proud in Beeston*. When they launched it, Adult Social Care bought copies to use as a training resource for staff. In addition to this, she had an article printed about BAFF's inclusive exercise group in the *Learning Disabilities Practise Journey*, Royal College of Nursing,

February 2011 edition. Baff2007@hotmail.co.uk

Kauser's achievements since she became involved with Carers Leeds and Carers UK have been many, including working with the School of Healthcare at the University of Leeds. Once a young girl of twelve, caring for her two brothers, who lacked confidence and was near to despair herself, she has risen to the challenges that caring brings, is now married with three adult children, and she is a confident and successful representative for carers. One of her many achievements was being invited to a special event at Lambeth Palace in London in connection with Carers UK.

*Qualities and Skills*

**Carer's CV for their loved one**

**Responsible for:**

**Health, all aspects of life including:** appointments; doctor's / dentist / hospital physical / hospital mental health /chiropody / hearing aids / spectacles; incontinence pads; repeat prescriptions

**Disability equipment:** medical equipment / commode / bath aids / stairlift / hoists / grip handles / perching stool / wheelchair / over-the-bed table

**Paperwork:** benefit forms / lasting power of attorney/best interest / advanced statements / wills / audits / reports / assessments / letters / care plans / carers assessments / reviews / care plans for care agencies / complaint letters

**Finances:** banking accounts / direct payments / deferred payments / social services / benefits / rent / arrears / debt loans / payments / credit cards / bills / invoices

**Utilities:** electricity / gas and water board / landline / mobiles / television / council / TV licence / insurances

**Housing:** report any problems if a tenant lives in a council property

**Care homes:** care plans / DNARs / relatives meetings / tidying resident's wardrobe / checking on clothes / new ones to buy

**Loved ones in their own homes:** cleaning / washing / ironing / shopping / administer medication / nurse injections / treatment at home by district nurses / maintenance of loved one's home / changing light bulbs / smoke alarms going off / TV stopped working / painting / decorating

**Skills and persona:** assertive when appropriate / approachable / caring / cheerful / cooperative / devoted / decisive / diplomatic / endurance / empathy / friendly / listening skills / organisational skills / open-minded / optimistic / observant / punctual / perseverance / practical / patient / polite / reliable / respectful / responsible / realistic / sensitive / sense of humour / thoughtful / trusting / tactful / unselfish / understanding

This list is by no means exhaustive. Add your own attributes to it, and keep it as it may come in useful when you need words to describe your role.

**Carer's Personal Profile**

Name: Kauser

Address: Yorkshire

Contact Details:

**Personal Profile:** I am a sister carer for my two disabled, adult brothers aged forty-eight and thirty-nine. Both brothers have microcephaly, epilepsy and challenging behaviour. I have been a full-time carer for twenty-two years and, during those years, I have worked with my brothers settling them into my home and working with professionals to prepare my brothers for as much of an independent life as possible outside day services in the community. I enjoy talking to students and sharing my expertise of caring with them. I feel valued, respected, and I am treated as an equal.

**Employment History:** nursery nurse officer. Twenty-two years of lived experiences being a carer. College of Social Work endorsement reviewer involved in the design, delivery and evaluation of qualifying social work education.

**Education and Qualifications:** the university of life and caring

**Voluntary Work:** community work in order to help people from all multicultural and diverse communities achieve a better quality of life through health groups and training. As a disabilities coordinator, I help develop new services for 'Health for All'. I am currently a care educator for Leeds University in all areas of learning and included in involvement advisory, steering and planning groups with lecturers at Leeds and Huddersfield Universities.

**Achievements:** Induction Award for supporting people with learning disabilities. Developed a community Action Group for Families which is a service user and carer-led community group.

**Hobbies and Interests:** When I get the opportunity, I enjoy walking, going to the cinema and reflexology.

**Groups:** member of: Social Work Team Practical Assessment Panel (PAP), Servicer User and Carers (SUC) strategy group Social Work Team, Public and Patient Involvement working group, Patient Carer Community (PCC), Involvement Advisory Group (IAG). I have also worked with student social workers and nurses and mental health nurses.

**Skills and Additional Topics:** writing scenarios, teaching, co-production presentation, interviewing, video interviews, planning meetings, programme management team, DVDs, digital stories and several articles. As a full-time, unpaid carer, I am responsible for all aspects of my brothers' care at home and at the day centre, in addition to all the paperwork in terms of sorting out and writing letters when problems and difficulties arise.

I guess the moral of this chapter is to never underestimate a carer.

Carers are:

- Doctors
- Mentors
- Social workers
- Advocates, appointees
- Parents
- Domestic helps
- Negotiators
- Diplomats
- Politicians
- Nurses
- Councillors
- Guardians
- Friends
- Confidants
- Lawyers
- Accountants
- Pharmacists

Carers have to have knowledge of:

- Health services
- Mental health
- Human rights
- Disability act
- Carers' rights
- Service users' rights
- Medication
- Treatments
- Mental Health Act
- Care assessments
- Care programme approach
- Benefits

Carers have to be:

- Precise
- Good communicators
- Good listeners
- Cool
- Calm
- Rational
- Knowledgeable
- Confident
- Patient
- Understanding
- Supportive
- Tolerant
- Compassionate
- Sensitive
- Constant
- Reliable
- Trustworthy
- Punctual

Add your own skills to this list. Use for discussion in 'Carer Involvement Groups.'

# CHAPTER 6

# Who Cares Anyway?

DISASSOCIATION BY FAMILY AND FRIENDS
WHO CARES FOR THE CARER?
COPING STRATEGIES

As a society, we talk much more about mental and physical health than we ever did, with a much more substantial and positive approach, however, when it comes to families and caring the story is quite different, as families can and do fall apart because they cannot agree with one another on subjects such as care, end of life, inheritance, choice of partner, addiction, illness and divorce.

## There's Caring and then there's Caring

*What do we mean by caring?*

**Caring is:** showing kindness, concern and loyalty, because someone who cares emotionally accepts you for who you are. They ask how you are, how your day has been, they really listen to you and give you help and support. They genuinely take an interest in you and your life with no hidden agenda.

*What is caring?*

**Caring is:** someone who cares for a person who is unable to look after themselves and gets paid for doing this work, and someone who does exactly the same work who does not get paid.

*How do we care?*

**Practical care:** is given in an abundance of ways, depending on the person you are looking after, and for many carers the physical side of caring can be extremely exhausting.

**Mentally and emotionally:** the paid worker is trained to do the physical job of caring, but one cannot do this without a certain degree of emotion and feeling for their patients in a variety of settings and circumstances. However, the only way I can describe the immensely deep feelings and thoughts that unpaid carers feel is to quote these words written by Sanober Khan, author and poet of *A Thousand Flamingos*: '*Sometimes I think, I need a spare heart to feel all the things I feel.*'

Someone who does not care demonstrates disinterest, is unmoved and unconcerned, along with being unfeeling and impervious.

**Disassociation by Family**

*What is dissociation and why does it happen?*

The disassociation talked about in this chapter is not to be confused with that of the dissociation of an individual with mental health difficulties, who distance from themselves and family. That kind of dissociation is the way that the mind copes with stress due to trauma, specific mental health problems, alcohol, medication and other mental or physical conditions.

During my years of caring, disassociation is not a subject that carers readily and openly talk about because it is too upsetting, it can be embarrassing or both, possibly giving the impression that the carer is struggling to cope. Some carers have conveyed their very sad stories of relationships breaking up because other members of the family cannot cope with the pain, stress and demands that caring entails. Several carers have commented that they do not get invited to family occasions because the assumption is that they will not be able to attend – but it would just be nice to be asked.

So what drives the sole carer to care yet drives other members of the family away?

Disassociation by family and friends can be what happens next when someone suddenly finds themselves in a caring situation and, at some stage, perhaps altercations from family raise their threatening, unpleasant and troublesome standpoints.

**SANE www.sane.org.uk**

SANE's observations are that families who find themselves in this situation of giving day-to-day care have:
- Very little training and support on how to embark on such a responsibility.
- They suggest that family members talk to each other in order to develop a practical and positive attitude.

- Ensure that all those concerned have the same understanding and position.
- Be understanding of everyone's circumstances and divide responsibilities according to strengths.

**www.Aplaceformom.com**

A Place for Mom reports their findings on some of the reasons for these divisions:

- When there is a fall out, carers can feel isolated, alone and resentful.
- If there is a disagreement about how much care is needed for an elderly parent, get an expert view.
- If one person is left to do all the heavy lifting.
- When one sibling excludes other siblings from decision-making.
- Past negativity in family life as a child.
- Parents resisting care.
- Arguments about paying for care, suggests establishing financial roles in advance.
- Different care opinions for end of life.
- When family members disassociate because you are an embarrassment to them with all the problems you have to deal with.

My own observations include:

- Living too far away to be able to do any caring on a regular basis.
- Other members of family say they have their own family to think about.
- One sibling having lasting power of attorney whilst the other siblings want it changed.

- Carers have stated that they are the sole carer because family members do not want to care or cannot cope with a caring role in terms of all aspects of illnesses.
- If the main caring role is falling to you, it may be that family can help in other ways in terms of giving you a break for a few hours through the day.
- Looking into what kind of respite is available for you and your loved one.
- Inheritance disputes.

As for the latter reason, as shocking as this may sound, it has been said family members who have had very little input, or none at all, in the caring role are usually the first ones to start taking charge of everything when their loved ones are at the end of life. Carers have stated that disputes occur over inheritance, even before a loved one's demise, as well as how monies or property will be divided. Suddenly quarrels from family members may arise with the main carer, in terms of them now wanting power and control, when one sibling already has power of attorney and another sibling wants it changed.

These kinds of issues cause so many family arguments and distress in a caring situation that perhaps some of these dilemmas can only be resolved by talking to the professionals, this might be family councillors, or lawyers that specialise in these matters, so it is useful to seek professional, constructive advice and guidance in these situations.

If it is possible though, talking together as family is usually the best option, with a view to looking at and discussing each other's skills and situations and how these could contribute in helping the main carer practically. For instance, if a family member can give their sibling two or three hours respite one afternoon week for them to take a break, this is a big contribution and always welcome. Just talking about each other's doubts, fears and anxieties can be eased together as a family, with or without expert guidance.

Our expectations of one another should be reasonable for all involved with their loved one, and yet again carers' helplines and carer support groups may be a big help in being able to talk about your experiences, in addition to listening and learning from other carers who have already walked down that road and who can help with problem-solving.

Many families pull together when caring is needed for a loved one, although I have lost count of the number of carers who have told me that they are the sole carer because family members do not want to care, or cannot cope with a caring role in terms of all aspects of illnesses. Numerous reasons are given, including living too far away to be able to do any caring on a regular basis, whilst others have their own families to think about. Carers have conveyed their very sad stories of relationships breaking up because one or other of spouses/partners cannot cope with the pain, stress and often demanding role that caring entails.

As if all that is not enough, situations are made worse for the carer when the problem is not of the carer's or family's making but very often from external agencies, leaving the carer to contend with the practicalities of something that should have been done/delivered/provided/or dealt with. This unproductive lack of action, along with nettlesome attitudes towards the carer, may result in the carer's mental health being exacerbated.

If you are a carer and feel alone, speak to your own local professionals and groups that can help.

## Dissociation by Friends

As carers we soon learn who our true friends are, don't we? Have you had friends who you always thought were good friends and then suddenly betray you? Friends who purported to support you and that you have built up a trust with, only to be utterly shocked and disillusioned when they take advantage of your situation and 'stab you in the back'. So-called friends that you genuinely took an interest in, supported them all the time with their personal problems and then, when you need help and a rafter of solidarity, it comes as a crushing blow when you are rejected, abandoned and never contacted again.

Some of this behaviour may possibly be through traits of jealousy, selfishness, bitterness and insecurity reasons known only to the offender when they do not tell us what is wrong. We then feel a deep hurt, betrayed, stitched up and let down by people who we thought were our friends, ethical, dependable and honourable, until we see their true colours. Perhaps the perpetrator never recognises a hurt they cause, and probably never takes the time to understand the situation. It is heartbreaking when families and friends cut ties or bury their heads in the sand, so forgive us carers for wanting the ostrich to make another hole so we can stick our heads in it.

People who on one hand demonstrate understanding, compassion and sympathy and then rescind it with the other are not uncommon, usually at a time, on that rare occasion when you really need their support, it is not forthcoming. Not that many carers ever want sympathy, because caring is not about that, but empathy is fine. A fake friend likes to hang out but wants all the attention on them, their interests and their needs, yet when we need help they are not willing to put themselves out. I have learned my lessons, through various experiences, and what to do in this situation and that is to sever ties and get on with life.

**Who Cares for the Carer?**

Is it your wife, husband, partner, both, brother, sister, daughter, son, uncle, aunty, extended family...?

Carers need support in terms of:
- Someone to talk to
- Respite
- Practical help
- Emotional support
- Professionals
- Family
- Friends
- Neighbours

**Coping Strategies**

These include indulging in a particular hobby, or trying new ones, such as taking a long, hot soak in the bath to soothe one's mind and body, relaxation techniques, yoga, in addition to making time to pop out for a coffee with friends, going to support groups, socialising with like-minded people in support groups and going out for the day.

I am not even going to try to write about all the coping mechanisms we hear about, because I believe these are very personal to the individual, and it really boils down to what you choose to do and how it fits in with a caring role. Organisations for carers often run courses on coping mechanisms with many carers reaping the benefits from them.

Is there enough help for you as a carer? If there is not then seek advice from professional organisations such as Age UK, Carers Trust, Carers UK, Carers Leeds or your local adult social services, as many of these organisations, and similar, have websites and helplines with information on a variety of topics. There will always be an expert in these matters that can give constructive advice and point you in the right direction to ensure your needs are met.

## Julie and Bev

*Scene: Julie and Bev at Julie's home sat on the sofa having a cup of coffee.*

"Right, listen to this then, Bev, according to this article, I can reduce my stress by avoiding caffeine."

"Oh right, that sounds good. Carry on then, I'm listening. Do you want a top-up?" she said holding the coffee pot in Julie's direction.

"Oh, yes please. Also avoid nicotine, pass us the ashtray, Bev, please," she continued, as the long, wavy shaft of ash floated into the tray. "Physical activity is good for reducing stress. Right, well I get enough of that when I am caring and on the go all day, running after the kids. Up and down the stairs, cleaning, moving the beds to move the rubbish that the kids have left there, to move the vacuum back and forth underneath. Lifting, running, walking, it never ends. I can't afford to go to a gym. Wouldn't want to, anyway, with all those slim, young lasses that go."

"You're not fat though, Julie, you're in proportion."

"No, I don't think I am, Bev, really. How can I be in proportion when a pair of size sixteen jeans is tight and an eighteen is baggy, what kind of proportion is that?"

"Well I think you always look good, Julie."

"That's what Mike says."

"Well believe him, because it's true. What else does the article say?"

"It says eat healthily. I try, but it's just not that easy. I'm too knackered to cook every night, so we end up eating fast food, I hate it. Anyway, it says also talk about your feelings. Well I do, I talk to Mike, and I talk to you, but you can bet your bottom dollar that in between talking I get broken off because the cat has just spewed a furball or one of the kids has.

"When the kids were in bed the other night, and Robby was settled, I thought I would take a lovely, long, relaxing bath, that's a relaxation technique. I was just going to pour my best scented bubble foam into the bath when I saw the biggest spider you have ever seen sitting there, just staring at me. I thought to myself, *Quick, swill it down the plughole with hot water*. Its massive eyes on its massive body stared at me as if it knew what I was thinking of doing to it, but it was way too big to be swilled down the plughole.

"My heart was racing, as I yelled downstairs for Mike. He came up the stairs like a thunderous pack of hippos, then I heard him trip, he does that when he tries to take the stairs two at a time."

"So," said Bev, as she shivered at the thought of this mighty spider, "what did Mike do with the spider then, Julie?"

"He caught it in a giant, empty pickled onion jar and let it go outside."

"It can't have been that big, Julie."

"Oh, you didn't see it, Bev, you didn't see it. It sort of took the edge off relaxing somehow. Kept thinking that the spider might have had a friend with it just lying in wait, ready to crawl up from the bath panel to see where its eight-legged, hairy friend had got to. Anyway, I thought I would catch up on some sleep by having an early night after my bath. I read my book for a while, fell asleep, then woke up with a hot flush three hours later."

"Know the feeling," said Bev, as she continued. "Does it give any more ideas?"

"Well," said Julie, "it just really finishes by telling me to manage my time, take control of my life, and don't let the big issues that crawl into one's life scare you." Julie and Bev burst out laughing.

"Well," said Bev, "you know what they say, laughter is the best form of medicine, and we can't argue with that one, can we?"

---

For me personally, relaxation is writing and singing with all my lovely friends in the choir. Their friendship is significantly valuable and rewarding; a group of ladies who are kind, compassionate, honest, helpful, gracious and non-judgemental, and just as important make me laugh. Singing releases endorphins, the feel-good factor, so the deep breathing and breath control exercises we do draws the oxygen into the blood thus resulting in better circulation and reduces stress. It is also said that it is an aerobic activity which is just as well, because my days of squats, lunges, crunches and bent-over row are long gone. Unwinding is essential, and my wonderful husband and I do this by chatting with a coffee, or sometimes a glass of wine in the evening, in a peaceful setting. His unsurmountable support and sense of humour sees us laughing, on numerous occasions, at sometimes silly, little things. Ah well, another day tomorrow.

# CHAPTER 7

# Engaging with Agencies

LIVED EXPERIENCES

THERE'S A FROG IN THE BASEMENT

WHAT NOW?

## Introduction: co-production theory and practice relevant to the role and experience of the carer and caree

It is highly likely that the most vulnerable people in society, along with organisations, are being affected in a climate of many changes, including the coronavirus pandemic, but even before the pandemic we have been faced with cutbacks, a lack of resources and crucial public services that have been distorted and sapped. So what is co-production and how do we implement it? First of all, the theory is said to be a set of statements or principles devised to explain a group of facts, along with co-production in social care which is defined by the Social Care Institute for Excellence (SCIE) as: *a meeting of minds coming together to find a shared solution [Think Local Act Personal]*, whilst practice is the actual implementation of an idea, belief or method.

*...a way of working whereby citizens and decision makers, or people who use services, significant others, family carers and*

*service providers work together to create a decision or service which works for them all. The approach is value driven and built on the principle that those who use a service are best placed to design it. [Skills for Health]*

This is an extremely valid and pivotal statement that is crucial, essential and necessary to all the issues that are raised in this book. Statements, principles and problems, along with the causes and effects on the carer practically, physically and mentally, are all emphasized in every Lived Experience.

It is hoped that the issues and barriers highlighted in these experiences will also encourage all organisations, government and corporate, to look more deeply into what services they provide, how they are provided and whether they support the carer in terms of training, development and education.

The keynote is discussion, working together, listening, sharing ideas and implementing the service and product which works for us all, therefore I reiterate that the approach is value driven and built on the principle that those who use a service are best placed to design it and in some cases that includes carers.

Engaging with Agencies covers the subtitles below:
- Health and Social Care
- Working Between and Across Government Departments
- Local Authority
- Care Homes
- Corporate Businesses

Each of these headings include:
- A Lived Experience

- A Personal Reflection
- There's a Frog in the Basement – Unexpected incidents that have to be dealt with as soon as possible
- What Now? – One problem follows another

Discussion points:
- After reading the experiences, discuss and list the issues arising.
- What have you learnt from any or all of these Lived Experiences?
- What has worked well?
- What can be done to improve the situation for the carer?

All of the Lived Experiences depicted throughout this book can be used for discussion and training purposes in the following sectors: business, student mental health nurses, student social workers in educational establishments such as universities or colleges, care support groups and community projects related to caring. The Perceptual Table in Chapter 9 is designed to highlight briefly how the issues depicted may affect the carer emotionally, physically, socially, spiritually and psychologically.

**All Hushed Up**

Not long after arriving home from the hospital with our new baby, a brother for our eldest son, I became concerned about a rash that Jay had developed from his waist down. Of course, at this stage, he had not been diagnosed with any of the other conditions mentioned earlier. He was constantly being sick and had diarrhoea. I was speaking to a friend of mine, on the phone, who had had her second baby around about the same time as

I had Jay. I told her about the rash on Jay's body. I discovered, from my friend, that her midwife had been taken off her regular caseload in order to deal with several other babies that also had these rashes. Sharon asked if I would like her to contact the midwife, on my behalf, to ask her to come to see Jay. Of course, I said I would appreciate a visit.

The following week, the midwife visited us and, after examining Jay, she confirmed that this rash was the same as the other couple of babies she had seen. The rash I was told was called pemphigus, a skin disease in which watery blisters form on the skin. She advised me to treat these blisters as one would with a burn which was to make sure that no covers were touching his skin when he was in the crib. Until such a time as the rash had completely cleared, I was not allowed to take Jay to the local baby clinic, therefore the midwife continued to visit us at home.

When Jay finally became well enough to go out, I took him to the baby clinic to have him weighed and checked and to see my health visitor.

Mrs Andrews welcomed us back and, during our conversation, she said, "Off the record, the pemphigus that Jay had, well, it was all a bit hushed up."

I asked her why. Apparently, there had been a stillbirth in the same delivery bed that I'd used, and possibly, because it had not been cleaned and sterilised fully, if at all, that is how he'd contracted it. I was already in the second stages of labour when I went into hospital, and it was a quick birth with only one nurse on duty, being Christmas it was a skeleton staff.

**Personal Reflection:** I was shocked to hear what my health visitor had told me, and did not really know what to say or do. The thought of investigating this incident further never really occurred to me at that time, as I was just so happy that my baby was now well.

It was only much later when I started to think about the situation and wondered more about the cause of the rash, as I only had the member of staff's word for it at that time. I wondered why a proper diagnosis of the rash was never confirmed by a doctor.

I remember feeling very isolated at the time, as we were never visited by any other professional except the midwife, and in addition to this, I was worried about this condition, anxious about the potential outcome and naïve as to what, if anything, I should do in a situation like this.

**Health and Social Care**

**Deprivation of Oxygen at Birth**

**Lived Experience 1 (1978)**

*"I am so sorry to tell you that your baby has been born with a deprivation of oxygen which has resulted in a cerebral palsy down his left side most likely resulting in him having special needs."*

That was just over forty-one years ago, yet it only seems like yesterday when I was given this news, and I had so many questions flying around in my head that I could not pin one of them down long enough to remember which one to ask the consultant first, other than, "What will the future be like for my son?" I guess it was a diagnosis that could not be given immediately at birth, it was only later, when Jay started to try to crawl, that we detected something was wrong.

Like all mothers, I watched my son with pride, as he crawled slowly across the lounge carpet; however, it was only seconds before it soon became apparent that he was not moving the way he should be. As Jay pulled himself along, he was dragging his left leg, in addition to having difficulty gripping anything with his left hand. Referring to my child development textbook for an answer as to why this was happening, I did not find any information that would help me, although to be fair, I am not sure what I was looking for in the first place.

I told the nurse about this on our next visit to the baby clinic, I am sure many of you remember the baby clinics and baby doctors as they were referred to back in1978, consequently the baby doctor made a referral to the hospital for Jay straight away.

After having had an initial visit with the professor at the paediatric hospital, it was not long before we were on our way for a second appointment to see the professor's understudy at a child development centre, and it was at this appointment I was told that Jay, due to a deprivation of oxygen at birth, had cerebral palsy affecting his left side. After a while, when my brain had adjusted to the news, I began to ask myself how and why this had happened, and then asked the consultant. I was told that it was just one of those things.

**Personal Reflection:** Possible reasons as to how this particular condition is caused:

- Lack of oxygen from the umbilical cord to the baby
- Possible inadequacy of foetal monitoring
- A lack of clinical knowledge
- A failure to follow guidelines
- Failure to ask for senior medical assistance
- Error in drug administration
- The most common cause – human error

Was this a failure to follow guidelines or was it an error? Should there have been further investigation as to what happened at the time of birth when a diagnosis of this nature is determined? Or do we settle for a 'passed off' statement, being 'It's just one of those things'?

**There's a Frog in the Basement:** I am in a meeting today and, although it can be quite a rush to get there, sometimes I really feel that I am contributing a fundamental and valid opinion of whatever it is we happen to be discussing from the carer's point of view.

"Apologies from Paul," said the chair. "He is dealing with a crisis with his son."

About an hour into the meeting, my phone buzzed. I got up to leave the room to answer it. This is never a problem when in a meeting, as everyone present know that carers must be contactable at any time of the day.

"Mum."

"Yes. Are you okay, Jay?"

"No, not really. Well, I'm okay, but there's a frog in the basement."

"What!"

"There's a frog in the basement."

"What? A real one?"

"Yes."

"Oh no. Well just shut the basement door, so it can't get up the cellar steps into the kitchen and room, and I'll see to it when I get back from the meeting."

There was a pause for a few seconds, along with a lot of moving, banging about and chuntering.

"What are you doing, Jay? Are you okay?"

A few seconds silence.

"Jay, are you okay?"

"I got it! I got it!"

"How did you get it?"

"I grabbed a cereal bowl and went into the basement and then followed it until it jumped into the bowl, and then I took it out into the garden and let it go."

"Oh, well done." Problem solved.

"But I think there is another one in there too."

**What Now?:** "We booked the taxi for 8.30 a.m. so what's happened to it?" I said to my husband. My dad, oblivious to what was going on due to severe Alzheimer's, sat in the wheelchair all ready and patiently waiting to go. The manager of the care home said she would ring to find out if the taxi was on its way.

"Yes," she said, "it's on the way. They said five minutes."

This was third time we had booked a wheelchair taxi for hospital appointments and again it was late. The journey to the hospital would take thirty minutes at best, and then we had to book in, go to the loo, not just Dad but me as well. The appointment was at 9.15. It was now five minutes to nine and the five minutes had now turned into fifteen. We were definitely going to be late now.

We decided we would take Dad in our car; however, this was difficult because of the massive, cancerous tumour on his leg and having to be so careful to lift him into the car. When carers have the discomfort of back problems, lifting is not the easiest task to undertake. Just as we got Dad into the car, the taxi turned up. I was very annoyed, to say the least.

"This is the third time you have been late to take us to a hospital appointment, and when you get here, you are not even a wheelchair taxi and you have not got the courtesy to even apologise. Forget it; I certainly will not be using your company again."

I know I am not the only carer to have experienced this scenario; it is quite simply down to people not listening and not being punctual. The carer is always thinking about the consequences of whatever eventuality arises and, in this case, it meant that being very late, we would have to go to the back of the queue, or even worse, the appointment would have to be rearranged.

---

**Health and Social Care**

**Hemiplegia**

**Lived Experience 2**

How hemiplegic children could be helped, in those days. The document below was given to me when Jay was approaching the age to start nursery school. It is written here verbatim from the original I was given and still have to this day.

**Help for Teaching Staff, if you have a young Hemiplegic Child entering your school.** (approx. 1981)

Hemiplegia or Hemiparesis, means a one-sided weakness, affecting the arm and leg of the same side. In some cases the arm is usually more affected than the leg. The weakness is due to a lack of development of the part of the brain which controls and coordinates the movements of the body. It is not due to a disorder of the muscles or nerves.

Occasionally these children will have a visual field defect on the same side of the body as the weakness, leading to a tendency to bump into things on the affected side. Learning difficulties [specific] are not uncommon, such as perceptual difficulties or short attention span, may also be present.

The arm and leg may show signs of tightness due to irregular muscle pull, the wrist, fingers, elbows and shoulder may be flexed. There will be variations of these symptoms depending on the severity of the condition. This condition may be helped and improved, but the disability will never be cured entirely and the child must be trained to live with this handicap and make the best of his potential.

There are various ways in which teachers and helpers in school can assist and guide but should also be aware of the physical problems these children have, in order to be able to foresee some of the pitfalls.

**Problems to be recognised and Pitfalls**

Problem: There may be a sensation loss on the affected side, partially affecting the hand.

Pitfall: Watch out for hot radiators, hot water taps etc.

Problem: There may not be normal balance reaction on the affected side.

Pitfall: If rushing in a crowd of children, or hurrying downstairs or tripping during P.E. [physical education]. He will not be able to save himself from falling, by putting out his arms as a normal reaction.

Note: – The use of the word 'he' on its own in this document is not politically correct in today's terminology, as this is usually written as he/she. The first recorded use of the term 'politically correct' is by Toni Cade Bambara in the 1970s, author of *The Black Woman*. [*Google*]

Problem: Due to a reduction of power in the arm, he may not be able to hold on to apparatus with two hands, during P.E. or carry objects one in each hand about the classroom.

Pitfall: He may fall from apparatus if unable to hold on with two hands. He will not be able to carry books and crayons, or other two objects about the classroom or playground and may find it difficult in carrying a dinner tray.

**Ways of helping**

Try to see, whenever possible, that the affected hand is open and when sitting on the floor it should be used as a prop, palm flat on the floor. Always use two-handed activities [ball games, plasticine etc.] the affected hand working as a helping hand; never push him to make it the leading one.

When writing or reading try to keep the hand on the desk, preferably holding the paper or book down, this keeps the body equal and prevents asymmetry.

If possible always sit on the hemiplegia side of the child, if you are sitting to work with him, so that he has to turn towards you, and thus make his weight distribution of his body equal, and also make him aware of that side. If taking him by the hand, always take the affected arm, bringing it forward to even up his posture.

## Discourage

1. Jumping from apparatus or any jumping exercises in P.E. because this stimulates his heel to rise and also make his arm rise in the air, bent at the elbow.

2. Sitting between his knees on the floor, always bring his legs forward so he is sitting firmly on his bottom.

School outings may be hazardous due to slow progress over rough ground and would need a member of staff to give help.

> **Personal Reflection**: At the time, this information was extremely useful to me, and the school, in addition to this, regular massage of his leg and arm to help with spasms of the limbs also helped. Although we were still in our early days dealing with Jay's condition, it was still a worrying time. Yes, we now knew his physical disabilities but, as yet, not his mental health. As parents, we just want do whatever we can for our children, and we quickly get into a routine of implementing whatever the doctor has said is needed, to help them, in our case it was the exercises and massage.

**There's a Frog in the Basement: It's Cold in Here** During the meeting, my mobile buzzed. I briskly walked out of the office to find somewhere quiet to answer it.

"Hello Jay, are you okay?"

"No, not really," he replied.

"Why, what's wrong?"

"The heating's not working."

[Inner thoughts] *It is summer and warmish.*

"Mum, are you still there?"

"Yes, yes, I'm here. Just trying to think what to do. Is Jenny still with you?" (Jenny is Jay's support worker.)

"Yes, but she doesn't know what to do."

"The only thing I can do is ring the housing when I get home and make an appointment for them to come and look at the boiler. Is that okay with you? I'll be home in about two hours. They will still be open then. Are you warm enough?"

"No."

"Okay. The fan heater is in the basement; put that on in the room. It will keep you going until I can sort something out. Are you okay with that?"

"Yes, okay."

"As far as hot water, you will have to boil a kettle for the time being. I will ring you when the meeting has finished."

"Okay. Thanks, Mum."

Back in the meeting. "Sorry about that." [Inner thoughts] *What were we talking about now?*

**What Now?:** I had just arrived at the hospital, eighty miles away, to see my mother who had recently had a stroke. I found myself liaising with a different health authority and, during a conversation with the social worker, I asked if she would be good enough to contact me in connection with all aspects of my mother's care, as I was the main carer for my parents.

The social worker said, "I do not class you as a carer."

"I beg your pardon?" I said. "I am very much my parents' carer. Have you never heard of long-distance caring and sandwich carers? We do exist."

---

**Health and Social Care**

**Injury to the Brain/Cerebral Palsy**

**Lived Experience 3**

It was only a few days before Christmas Day when I went into labour, and the festive celebrations were well underway. Whether it was because of Christmas, or for some other reason that there was limited staff on duty in the maternity hospital, it resulted in there being only one midwife on duty throughout my labour and childbirth, and I was already in the second stages of labour when I arrived at the hospital so it was a quick birth and, as I described earlier, Jay was diagnosed with cerebral palsy.

*Cerebral palsy is a group of disorders that affects movement and muscle tone or posture caused by damage that occurs to the immature brain as it develops, most often before birth. Signs and symptoms appear during infancy or preschool years.* – [] This condition can also be caused by an injury to the brain, before, during, or shortly after birth.

Brain damage resulting in cerebral palsy can occur in pregnancy, during labour and delivery, shortly after birth or something that goes wrong during gestation or birth. [*Birth Injury Help Centre www.birthinjury helpcentre.org*] Whatever the reason, any one of the above, for parents it generates questions, in my case it was just one of those things. Do I have to accept that it was just 'one of those things'?

As a result of this diagnosis, I took Jay several times a week, over a number of years, to the hospital for assessments, speech therapy, occupational therapy, physiotherapy and educational psychology. In addition, there were many meetings with the social worker, and I could not fault the team's professionalism at the hospital, in terms of the support and care they gave us, and I got to know a lot of the mums and their wonderful children there.

One day, they were all talking about 'Attendance Allowance', which was once an allowance one could apply for, for a sick child. I did not know much about benefits at that time. One of the mums had a little girl, around the same age as Jay, who had exactly the same condition, for whom she claimed Attendance Allowance.

Helen said, "You ought to apply for the allowance, it really helps." So I did. My first application was dated May 1982, and an assessment was carried out by a doctor on Jay at our home.

The Department of Health and Social Security wrote to say '*that the Attendance Allowance Board had considered my claim and have noted the amount and sort of help required, but have decided that this attendance does not satisfy the conditions which are laid down by law,*' concluding their letter by apologising for sending me a disappointing reply.

I wrote a letter of appeal which resulted in another doctor visiting us to do a second assessment on Jay. The allowance was refused again. I was more upset and annoyed with the doctor's report, as it was full of inaccuracies and came across as belittling my child's condition; therefore, this certainly was not a true reflection on Jay's condition. I scrutinised this report, and made notes, which took many hours of hard work. After my personal cross-examining of the independent doctor's medical assessment, I wrote again, in an attempt to highlight the flawed and 'wide of the mark' report, in terms of the reality of Jay's condition.

My first question to myself was, *How was Helen granted the allowance for Trudy when her child had exactly the same condition as Jay, who was no worse, or no better than Helen's little girl?* In order to answer this question, I needed some professional legal advice. I rang a solicitor specialising in such matters and explained the situation. This is what he said to me.

"Had you given birth to a girl, they would have authorised the Attendance Allowance." He went on to say, "I would drop all my cases now to take this to court in terms of discrimination." He was prepared to take my case on, however, the only barrier

I had from going any further with this issue was the lack of money to pay legal fees; of course I could not afford to take this to court. Maybe these days it would be a different scenario. I hope it is.

I did, however, get in touch with my local newspaper which resulted in my local MP contacting me. He said he had seen the distressing story in the paper, about the need for help to look after my son, and went on to say that he would quite happily make representations on my behalf regarding this issue if I so wished. Needless to say, I accepted his offer of help, and he then consequently wrote to the Health Secretary of the time.

In October 1984, I received a reply from my MP and the Health Secretary. In the MP's letter he said, '*the answer from the Health Secretary seems to say 'Yes' you do need help to look after Jay, but it is not sufficiently marked to fall within the present law. You must consider what further action you want to take within the existing law and how we might together spotlight the need for better provision.*'

The Health Secretary's letter stated that he had referred to the medical comments I'd made in my letter, which I said had been ignored, and this was passed to the Board's delegate in which he stated that he acknowledged the comments and that they had been considered along with all the other evidence. In addition, the Health Secretary stated that the Attendance Allowance was being refused owing to not meeting the tick-box assessment and I could appeal.

His reply was not constructive or encouraging, and I felt that there was an injustice here with which I could not proceed. I was naïve about what I could do next but, without finances and support, the answer was 'not much'. This injustice was to be the instigator of the many social injustices, throughout mine and Jay's life, for me as a mother and carer looking after my baby with no idea as to what his future mental and physical well-being would be. A journey that would lead me into the world of caring and its many injustices, not just for us, but to try and be a voice for other carers as well, in order to speak out and make these wrongs right.

> **Personal Reflection:** I felt that in this lived experience there was an element of discrimination and that I had not really been listened to. Looking back on all these inequalities that I have dealt with over the years, I can only assume that they have happened for a reason, probably to prepare me for the biggest injustice that was yet come.

**There's a Frog in the Basement: Mission Impossible** My day begins at 6.15 a.m. when I take my tablets half an hour before I can have a cup of tea. I get up, shower, dress, don't really want anything for breakfast but know I have to eat, so I settle for a yogurt and banana followed by a speedy cup of coffee, whilst I have a quick recap on what I am going to be doing today.

*Ah, yes the council are coming any time between 8.30 and 1 p.m. to do a repair at Jay's.* As I log that thought, along with other mental notes for the day, in my mind, 'Mission Impossible' summons me to respond to my phone, as always, with a positive frame of mind. I swiftly swipe the phone to answer, because no mission can ever be impossible for a carer, it's just damned hard work.

"Hello Jay, you're up early. Are you okay?" I ask.

"Yes, I'm okay. What time did you say the council were coming?"

"Between 8.30 and 1 p.m."

"Okay, are you coming up?"

"Yes, just as soon as I'm ready, but I will be at yours for 8 a.m."

Before I set off, I make the bed, put the washing in the machine, and check Jay's accounts to make sure he is not overdrawn, check I have his daily medication to take up to him and leave the house at 7.40, calling at the shop for some bits and pieces for him. Just as I am walking back to the car park 'Mission Impossible' signals my response once again.

"Hello." It's Janice.

"You won't believe this," said Janice. "My washer has packed in, and I need some money to pay for it mending now because the repairman is coming in an hour."

Janice is the daughter of one of my relations, but since she lost her mother some years ago, I have been her guardian. She suffers with bipolar and has a dependency on certain substances, her way of self-medicating.

"When did the washer break, Janice?" I asked her.

"Just now," she said.

"So how come you've managed to get someone to come and see it so quickly then?"

"It's a friend. I phoned him, and he's coming over. Please can you lend me £40.00?"

"You haven't paid back the £20.00 I lent you a fortnight ago. What have you done with your benefit?"

I knew it would be the same old story, as she said, "It's just gone on the leccy and gas, and some on my phone. Please can you come up now or not?"

"Janice, you just expect me to drop everything, and never give me any warning. I'll come up now and, after this, Janice, I am not helping out financially again. I just can't afford to." I make a quick call to Jay to let him know I will be a few minutes late. "Jay, I have to go to Janice's. I won't be long."

"Okay," he said. "What's wrong now?"

"Tell you when I get back."

I am always prepared to deal with the unexpected demands of the day, but when I get calls like this from Janice they really stress me out, because I know deep down that what she has told me is probably a lie and, more than likely, the truth is that she needs money for something else.

Janice's illness can be very bad at times, however, when she is stable, she is a lovely girl with an excellent, creative talent and great fun to talk to, it's just that these situations are frequent, upsetting and frustrating, and I feel isolated in these circumstances due to my reluctance and embarrassment to talk about it. It is a different kind of caring to the care Jay needs and appreciates. I know full well that it is only Janice herself, along with professional support, which can give her the help she needs. On numerous occasions, she has tried to engage with services but always to no avail.

Back to Jay's, with not even time for a coffee, as the repairmen turn up just as I arrive. When they have finished, just over an hour later, I start the cleaning, make some lunch, or we go out for fast food. Back to Jay's, after calling at the shops again and the cash machine for him to get his money. I don't rush these errands, as I enjoy our time together, and if it is a nice day, we have a walk in the park. I enjoy our chats and, because of his witty and impromptu sense of humour, we have some good laughs. He is a very loving, placid and good-natured young man who, despite his difficulties, very often stills my troubled mind.

I arrive home at teatime and continue the washing after a cuppa with my husband, who has been busy with other chores in the house, and in the evening I try to get on with some paperwork. The report and audit for the Office of the Public Guardian (OPG) has to be tackled, as the deadline rapidly approaches. As I think about that task, I open the post and read the letter from the council saying they are thinking of withdrawing the parking permits in my son's area. My inner thoughts say, *Great that is all I need. If they do that, how on earth will I find a parking space near enough to carry the laundry and shopping bags back and forth?*

The parking permits are invaluable, so I immediately write an email to the councillor named on the letter inviting residents to get in touch should we have any queries, after I jot down some quick notes and questions about the issues. I will ask them exactly what is happening about this situation, and I would like to know if there has been a consultation with residents about this idea, which the letter seemed to suggest there had. If this is the case, why haven't we been informed? There will be service users who live on their own, and organisations should be aware that they may not be able to get to meetings on their own, in addition to those who have carers who need to be informed too so they can attend meetings such as this together. Both parties should have the opportunity to give their views on changes in their areas that may affect daily routines.

I conclude my email by stating that if the permits are going to be withdrawn, it will open the floodgates for anyone and everyone who does not live in the area to park in the bays, leaving residents with cars to park in already limited parking bay space.

This is an area that already experiences parking problems, and I would be most grateful that if this plan is implemented, you would give serious consideration to giving us some disabled parking bays for service users and carers like myself.

I receive a reply the same day, which I sort of half expected, as the councillor in question is a professional and compassionate individual and has dealt with many issues successfully. I was told that my concerns would be considered. This is work in progress.

**What Now?:** After everything was done and dusted at Jay's, I went to see Mum in the care home; she will be ninety-three this year. My husband and I sat in the communal lounge with her. She suffers with dementia/Alzheimer's, has lost the sight in one eye and can barely hear; therefore the following conversation was loud.

"Are you okay, Mum?"

"Yes, thank you, I'm okay. Is the family okay?"

"Yes, they are all okay. The chiropodist was supposed to be coming to see you today, wasn't he?"

"Who?"

"The chiropodist."

"I didn't hear what you said."

Elongating the words, I said, "The chirrr-opppo-dissst, you know, the man who does your feet."

"Oh yes, him."

"Did he come to see to your feet today then?"

"Who?"

"The chirrr-opppo-dissst, you know, the man who does your feet."

"Oh yes, he's been."

"How are they now then?"

"What was that love?"

"Have you got your hearing aids in, Mother?" I said pointing to her ears.

"No, can't be bothered with them. Too faffy."

I said, "How are your feet now then?"

"I don't really know, I've not had them that long."

After returning home, our late lunch at three thirty in the afternoon is a quick snack of Mini Cheddars and a Babybel cheese. One's mind is so busy, I find myself doing and saying silly things, like today for example, when I decided to have a banana sandwich, I went to the fridge and grabbed the cucumber from it.

"Have you seen the size of this banana?" I said to my husband. We just burst out laughing.

Looking forward to sitting down to watch TV and unwinding for an hour whilst eating this splendid feast of cucumber sandwiches accompanied by a tube of Pringles, it did not go according to plan due to quite a few interruptions including the phone. It took me nearly two hours to watch a four-month-old recorded episode of *Location, Location, Location*, therefore I did not really get the chance to appreciate the very expensive

Victorian five-bedroomed, three-bathroomed house with original features, situated on a six-acre plot, boasting a beautiful garden with well-established trees, that people do purchase whilst others can only dream of. My thoughts of chilling out with the reality of a practical *Escape to the Country* are now even thwarted by Covid.

---

**Health and Social Care**

**Managing a Disability**

**Learning to manage and grow with a disability**

**Lived Experience 4** (Approx. 1981-1983)

Now with an established routine of regular visits to the hospital two to three times a week, I was already educating myself in terms of finding out as much as I could about Jay's condition and how it would affect him.

Home computers entered the market in 1977, becoming more common in the 1980s and mainly used for games and word processing, however, I did not have the luxury of owning one, although the concept of tapping a little button to access instant information on the subjects I wanted appealed to me.

In my youth, I trained as a qualified touch, speed and audio typist, and in order to do that we had to use a typewriter on which the keyboard was devoid of its entire letters. It took me a long time to get used to the idea that, at some point, I would probably have to get a home computer. It was my sister that introduced me to them, as I was doing a lot of writing at the time and when I finally learnt how to use it I reluctantly said goodbye to my electric typewriter. Previous to that, most of the information I needed was given to me from the staff at the hospital.

I cared and helped Jay with the physical exercises he needed to do at home, including speech therapy, in between the regular visits to the hospital. I was always told to hold his left hand whenever walking with him, in order to increase the strength in his grip. His cerebral palsy affects the whole of his left side, so physical exercise is important to help improve strength, flexibility and balance, along with regular massaging of hands and legs to relieve spasms and tightness in muscles. Jay always seemed to benefit from this treatment and, even today, I still do that if he needs me to.

It is important to encourage finer motor skills when a child tends to use only the thumb and forefinger, making tasks like picking things up and fastening buttons much harder. His balance is also unsteady, and on one occasion, when I took my son to the general hospital, I was questioned about the bruises on Jay's arms and legs which were due to him falling a lot. I had never given them a second thought, however, the staff at the hospital thought differently and asked me all sorts of questions which seemed to, allegedly, accuse me of causing the bruises. I told them that Jay fell a lot due to his unsteady balance and gait problems when he was playing in the garden, and that they were most certainly jumping, very high, to incorrect conclusions, to the point where I felt intimidated and extremely upset.

For a mother, the guilt is bad enough when one's baby is born with a disability, we feel that we are the cause of our child's disability, and I asked myself if I had done something wrong whilst I was pregnant, if I did, what was it? I always ate healthily and looked after myself.

Whenever Jay attended his little friends' parties, I had to ask parents not to give him a glass (throwaway plates and cups were not as popular as they are these days) but a plastic cup, just in case he fell with it in his hand. In order to prevent accidents when your child has a disability, it is imperative that other adults responsible for your child's care on happy and fun celebrations such as this are informed of your child's needs, just as it is when a child has allergies to certain foods.

The resources I needed for Jay, such as a non-slip mat for the high chair tray, and table, specially designed knife and fork and many more aids, I was able to access from a disability centre. In addition, the hospital referred him to a shoe specialist where he was fitted with bespoke, little boots that were designed to support his ankles; they were pretty cool and looked just like any other kid's boots.

When Jay reached school age, there was a lot of debate about which school he should attend and the multidisciplinary team of professionals discussed special educational needs schools and mainstream school. It was decided that Jay attended mainstream school on the condition that he would be monitored and reviewed regularly.

The staff at the school were fully informed about Jay's condition and, although there was no such role as a special educational needs coordinator (SENCO), or support assistant, in mainstream school those days (1981), the staff were understanding and supportive and followed his regime.

One night, when Jay was in the bath, he said, "Mummy, why do the children call me names? Is it because I've got a funny hand?"

Trying to hold back tears, I said, "Don't take any notice of them. Just because you struggle a bit with your hand and leg, you are still as good as them and, even more, you're a very special, little person to me."

I was, of course, concerned about what Jay had told me, and the next day I had a word with the head teacher about this. She said she would bring this to the attention of her staff and would explain to the children that using cruel words to someone with a disability was not acceptable. I was beginning to wonder whether Jay might have been better at a school that would understand his needs more fully.

In 2013, approximately seven years ago, sometime during the summer, we were having a coffee at the shopping centre, and I got chatting to a young woman with a baby. We talked 'babies' in general at first, what was her name, how much did she weigh, when was she born, all the usual and exciting new baby talk mums have.

Although she was a few months old at the time, I was holding her little hand, when Mum said, "She was born with a lack of oxygen, causing cerebral palsy, affecting her right side."

As soon as she said that, I was immediately transported back to all those years ago when I was told exactly the same thing, and thoughts of my journey with Jay flashed through my mind and the unfamiliar journey about to face this new mum.

"It was difficult and upsetting telling my family and friends," she said. I had felt the same way.

We talked about caring and the support available, and I told her about Carers Leeds. She had not heard of them before, so I pointed her in right direction. She welcomed the helpful information I gave her. We talked about benefits, as she went on to say that she had applied for benefits to help her with the extra costs connected with caring, however this was denied, because the DWP said 'You are a mum and you would be caring for the baby anyway'. The very same thing happened to me forty years ago, why is this still happening? I wished her all the very best for the future and hoped all went well for her baby. I still wonder to this day how they both are now.

---

**Personal Reflection:** A baby diagnosed with cerebral palsy, or any other physical or mental health disability, is obviously going to have more needs and require extra care and support than a baby blessed with a clean bill of health.

So why, when applying for a benefit such as this, are we told, you are a mother and will be caring for the baby anyway?

---

Who knows what needs a child may require in terms of medical resources and equipment as it grows and develops, bringing with this care extra costs such as making regular visits to the hospital.

For some parents, these visits may consist of overnight stays or longer, along with constant lifelong care for other children; these families who are separated in such situations, find that being away from home brings its own strains and tensions. Constant anxiety and worry over finances and employment are always at the back of one's mind, but our main focus is obviously always on our child.

In some cases, each stage of a baby's development will unravel the truth of a child's real needs and care, to a greater or lesser degree, and as parents, we worry about whether our child's condition will improve, stay the same or get worse.

The medical term 'spastic' came into use to describe cerebral palsy. The Spastics Society, an English charity for people with CP (cerebral palsy) was founded in 1951. The word spastic was often colloquially abbreviated to shorter forms such as 'spaz'. A BBC survey ranked the word spastic as the second most offensive term for the disabled, just below 'retard' [*Wikipedia*]. When educating children or young people on disabilities (disabilities meaning mental or physical disability) it is much better to use the proper name of the disability (i.e. cerebral palsy).

A suggestion for a group activity/discussion would be to make a list of the more politically correct words we use today and compare them with the derogatory word list. It certainly highlights the way society's behaviour and attitudes have changed.

Derogatory Words

- Cripple
- Dumbo
- Handicapped
- Idiot
- Imbecile
- Mental

- Nutter
- Crazy
- Bonkers
- Retard
- Lunatic
- Maniac

Discussion

- Do we still witness any stigma to a child's physical or mental health in school?
- What support is given?
- What does that support look like now?
- How do parents explain to their child with a disability, and any other siblings, about this condition?

In my very early days of going into teaching, I needed to acquire some teaching practice, so a friend of mine who was already a special educational needs teacher arranged for me to go into the school she taught at, in order teach a small group of children who had many and various learning difficulties and behavioural problems.

We played games and chatted together and, one day, I undertook some very simple baking with them, the aim being to stimulate their young minds in an activity that was not too taxing but yet practically and creatively engaging, so what could be better than to rustle up some chocolate crispy buns?

In order to ensure that each of my six charges participated in this activity, I decided that they take it turns to put the ingredients into the bowl, and repeat the turn taking as we melted the chocolate, which took a little longer as the flame on the one-ringed stove was minimal.

One little boy, Billy, who was very funny and talked non-stop, I soon discovered he had no patience at all.

He said impatiently, "Miss, when is it my turn to stir?"

"Soon, very soon, Billy," I replied. "You went first last time, and there's only Janet to stir now and then it is your turn."

Janet, however, was stirring very slowly and overly precisely, when Billy, now fed up of waiting, suddenly blurted out, "Who wants to make ****** chocolate crispy buns, anyway?" Despite their problems, which made heart ache, they were good kids, and I really enjoyed my time with them.

During the 1990s, I joined the team of staff at a day and boarding school teaching drama and performing arts throughout the curriculum, along with drama therapy for statemented pupils who presented with Asperger's, ADHD, dyslexia and other difficulties.

Working with the special educational needs coordinator and educational psychologist following a pupil's assessment, we discussed the various needs of the child. For example, if a child had concentration problems, constantly fidgeting, interrupting and disrupting, a lack of focus, hyperactivity, obsessions, and speech difficulties, to name but a few, it was my role to focus and devise a bespoke learning programme that covered their needs. In addition to the difficulties already mentioned, body language, behaviour, eye contact, protocol and social skills was an essential part of this timetable in order to meet the needs of that particular child.

The SEN unit was a welcoming establishment within the school, and we all worked together as professionals, including working with parents. Our aims and objectives were to implement these programmes successfully, in order to achieve the pupil's full potential, where the vast majority of pupils, I am pleased to say, excelled.

Our productions, I will never forget, were momentous moments for us all, the pride and delight I felt for these very talented performers will always live in my memory. Rehearsals were a combination of amusement, silliness, laughter, dedication, commitment and hard work all coming together, as they stood on the stage, to give captivating performances of the various musicals we staged.

It was extremely rewarding to see their skills and talents emerge with a new-found confidence that would stand them in good stead in their years ahead. It was an honour and a privilege to teach at this school, and I am left with wonderful memories of all the performing arts pupils from year two right through to sixth form. You could say it was a class act.

*Imagination is everything. The potential possibilities of any child are the most intriguing and stimulating in all creation.* – Ray L. Wilbur Third President Stanford University

*It is the supreme art of the teacher to awaken joy in creative expression and knowledge.* – Albert Einstein

**Mental Health**

In the late 1950s and 1960s, we would never have seen television adverts on mental health, telling us that it is okay to talk about how we feel. Then Time to Change was formed in 2009 by mental health charities Mind and Rethink Mental Illness aiming to reduce health-related stigma and discrimination.

I was involved with Time to Change in Leeds, which was led by Tricia Thorpe of the Leeds and York Partnership Foundation Trust (LYPFT). The project we were involved in was called the human library. Many service users and carers, with different lived experiences on mental health, volunteered to take part in this initiative, they being the books. Events for the human library were arranged by Tricia and, on the day of the activity, the attendees were given a list of all the books available, they could choose several, and with a time limit on each one, we, as human books would speak to the participant about our lived experience on that particular subject, needless to say mine was on caring.

**Mental Health Hospitals**

Well known for her amazing photographs of the old High Royds Hospital in Guiseley, Leeds, Tricia published a book entitled *Laying Demons to Rest* depicting the yesteryear of the hospital with some stunning photos of the place.

**My personal story of High Royds**

Set in its own peaceful and tranquil grounds, High Royds was the perfect environment for rest and recuperation. I have been to the hospital on many occasions for the following reasons: as a mother visiting my son, as he started his journey towards healing; as a middle manager for the health service; and, when I left the NHS to go into teaching as a lecturer in further education, I went to High Royds again where I had the privilege of teaching some courses there.

My own personal feeling was one of awe when I first saw this large, Gothic complex of stone buildings, a splendid, beautiful, iconic building, surrounded by expansive, well-landscaped gardens and woodland and was opened in 1888 and known as the West Riding Pauper Lunatic Asylum, designed by architect, J. Vickers Edwards.

I could possibly put my gut feelings and recollection of my first visit in 1995 to this building down to my vivid imagination, or my sixth sense, because as I stepped inside this phenomenal hospital, I sensed a certain atmosphere, a combination and contrast of a few mixed feelings at the same time. One of eeriness and the other of calmness, and the whole ambience of this psychiatric institution gave me a feeling of positivity, hope and being 'free from stresses', yet at the same time I saw darkness, felt a sadness, sombreness and a despair that I suspect would not be far from the truth from what some of the patients felt and went through during their time there.

Although this was a fully functioning hospital, I strongly felt, perhaps, the underlying presence of the spirits of the sick people who lived there many years ago. Throughout my visits and work at the hospital, I invariably had to walk from one place to another via the vast and deserted corridors. There was one corridor, in particular, that I used regularly. It was eerily silent and always left me feeling a bit sick and, to be quite honest, just wanting to sit down and go to sleep.

The first time I walked down this corridor, I immediately detected a strange smell like ether which, research tells me, has a sweet smell and is mildly pungent, however, the vapour I caught was a distinctive yet faint smell that resembled the rubber mask I had put over my face if I had to have an anaesthetic at the school dentist.

One of the staff, who had worked there for a long time, showed me round and, as she did, told me that the patients of that era lived on the wards but had to work for their keep by working on the farm, in the kitchens, or in the laundry.

The building housed its own ballroom, cinema, post office, shop, hairdressers, library and butchers as well as dairies, upholsters, bakery, cobblers, surgery and dispensary. I remember the shop and post office were still there when I used to visit in the 1990s.

Some of these institutions have been described as prisons for the insane, and many of the patients never left them. Some of the treatments used were convulsive therapy, occupational therapy and hydrotherapy, but this was not in a pool as they are today, their hydrotherapy consisted of having to have continuous baths for hours and even days.

I know I am not the only one to pick up on certain atmospheres, smells and vibes from historical buildings, or to visualise and imagine what life was really like for these patients all those decades ago. Research tell us that hexafluoride was an inhalant used in psychiatric treatment in those days, in addition to hexafluoride I have no idea what other gasses were used, and I am not a scientist, however, as true as the rain falls from the sky, I smelt that smell.

**Managing a Disability:** Research studies show that babies who have complications at birth, which were premature or starved of oxygen (hypoxia), have an increased risk of developing the symptoms of psychosis. Researchers speculate there may be subtle changes in the brain's development because of hypoxia. Other research studies state the same, but also add that exposure to viruses or infections in the womb or early infancy may also have an effect. Jay was later diagnosed with schizophrenia due to the complications at birth.

**Personal Reflection:** The anguish and uncertainty of my son's health from birth to date has never left me, along with the constant worry and inconclusiveness of life for Jay, now and in the future.

As carers, we naturally support, care, talk, advise, guide and help in whatever we can and in whatever situation we are faced with, in addition to making ourselves heard when dealing with problems and injustices. We have to rely on the professionals to ensure that all medical and other information they have on our loved ones is detailed and accurate, because if it is not, just one wrongly written word or sentence could be misconstrued by another professional, resulting in the wrong medication and/or information on an assessment that portrays a totally false impression of the individual.

**There's a Frog in the Basement: Disappeared** "Mum?"

"Yes, it's me. Are you okay, Jay?"

"No, not really."

"What's wrong?"

"I can't find my door keys, and Jenny will be here soon. I can't let her in."

"Where did you last have them?"

"They were in the room and now they have just disappeared, everything just disappears in this house."

Reassuring Jay I said, "Okay, not a problem. I'll come up and help you look for them."

Lots of items have gone missing in Jay's house, some of them we find and some we don't. I was with Jay one day when he dropped one of the small remote controls on the floor, we immediately looked down at the floor and it was nowhere to be seen. Thinking it had slipped under the sofa, we lifted that up, but it wasn't there. It really was a mystery, the remote had just disappeared. I would not have believed it, had I not seen it myself. When a person with mental health problems relays incidents like this in conversation to someone else, or about an event in their life which can seem unbelievable, don't underestimate or make fun of them, it is probably true.

When I had a spare moment, I decided to google 'things that

go missing'. I was amazed to see just how many people had experienced the same events, so having read about other people's experiences, I was then able to reassure Jay that he was not the only one it happens to, nevertheless, we never did find the remote.

No one knows your loved one, the person you are caring for every day, as well as the carer does. I know all about my son and his life's journey, the places he's been on holiday, the days out, the sightseeing, the people and famous people he has met, courses he has been on, the joy and happiness we shared when he passed his driving test and got his first job. So if Jay ever tells you that he met Eric Pollard (Chris Chittell, *Emmerdale*) and Val Pollard (Charlie Hardwick, *Emmerdale*) as they say on *Would I Lie to You?*, it is true.

**What Now?:** I am dealing with two major official complaints at the same time, at the moment, and I am now suffering with extreme anxiety, feeling utter frustration and at screaming point. One of these complaints is to a hospital and the other to social services, both connected to the other complaint and still ongoing over three years later.

Have you encountered any of these problems?
- Making a verbal and/or written complaint.
- Ringing people to sort out various enquiries like problems with bank statements, other finances, benefits.
- Written emails because that is the only option one is given when there is no contact number, change an appointment, sort out paperwork, and try to resolve a mistake.

Why does it take so long to deal with these things? And how

many hoops have you had to jump through to get a solution, if any?

Have you ever had replies like these?

*She's on sick.*

*He's left.*

*She's retired.*

*He's on leave.*

*She's on maternity leave.*

*He's moved to another department.*

*Leave a message and we will get back to you.*

*We don't take messages, you will have to ring back when he is in.*

*Sorry, there is no one to take a message at the moment.*

*He's on paternity leave.*

*We don't deal that with that here.*

*The department has moved.*

*That service has closed down.*

*We don't do that any more.*

*It's delayed because of the Christmas break, summer holidays, Easter, bank holidays...*

*Sorry she's now left for the day* (at 2 p.m. in the afternoon).

*Sorry we have a backlog of work at the moment.*

*You really need to speak to the supervisor, but she is on holiday.*

*It's with our legal team at the moment.*

*The system is down, and we don't know how long for.*

*He's not in the office today.*

*She only works Tuesday and Wednesdays.*

*We don't have anyone else to deal with this; she's on long-term sick.*

*The computers have crashed.*

*It's delayed because we have a backlog of work.*

*She's not in the office at the moment. Can you ring back in half an hour?*

*I'll try to sort it out for you.*

*I'll pass the message on.*

*Can I get her to call you back?*

*You should have received that by now.*

**How much longer do I have to wait?**

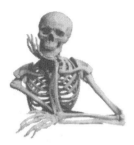

---

**Health and Social Care**

**Mental Health/Psychosis**

**Lived Experience 5**

**'Get out of the house, Mum, before he gets here.'**
(Approx. 1998-999)

It was a weekend, mid-afternoon, and I was sat on the sofa enjoying a quick cup of tea, when Jay came rushing in through the door frantic with worry. He grabbed my hand and was pulling me up from the sofa, at the same time begging me to get out of the house before the man got here to kill me.

I had to think very quickly about what to do to help Jay, knowing he had severe psychosis. Jay really believed this incident was going to happen.

"Okay," I said. "Let me just get my bag, and we will go for a drive in the car." My inner thoughts being, *It is a Saturday, who is around to help?* His dad was away and his stepdad also out for the day. I remained extremely calm and rational whilst my heart was thwacking against my chest, not because I was scared, but because my son was in so much distress.

The best thing to do at this moment was to go for a drive and talk, so we drove around for over four hours whilst chatting and reassuring him. Eventually, through tiredness, I pulled over and parked up.

"What are you stopping for, Mum?"

"So you can have a ciggy, and I can have a five-minute break from driving." After a long talk with Jay, comforting, supporting and reinforcing that we were both safe, I asked Jay how he was feeling.

"Not too bad," he replied.

"Do you want to go back home?"

Jay had calmed down and said he would like to do that. He was nearly eighteen when he had his first episode of psychosis. The psychiatrist stated that before a diagnosis could be made, Jay had to present three times with the same symptoms, and it was only after a further two crises, he was diagnosed with schizophrenia. Hospital admission was frequent from then on, sometimes by a section under the Mental Health Act, sometimes voluntarily.

**Personal Reflection**: Psychosis is a loss of contact with reality and is a symptom of a number of mental illnesses rather than a medical condition in its own right. A severe psychotic episode in which things are happening is very real to the person experiencing it.

When I witnessed a psychotic episode for the first time, a million thoughts were racing around in my head about what to do. Because mental health is more talked about now, professionals in this field help carers to understand this particular symptom and what to do in a crisis. However, twenty plus years ago, information was not as detailed as it is today, and everyone's experiences are different. Carers have to think on their feet, have to stay calm. I could not even begin to imagine how my son was feeling, but I was going to try, try very hard, to get a better understanding of how I could help him.

As well as many other aspects, psychosis can increase a person's sensitivity, leaving them feeling extremely frightened and overwhelmed. Understanding psychosis and having a crisis plan is essential, and as carers we can help in these situations by keeping our loved ones safe by giving them emotional support, demonstrating compassion, understanding and listening to them. Respect their wishes, speak calmly and offer suggestions and options about what you can do to help, and get professional advice.

A carers' role comes to a temporary stop when a crisis happens, because it is at this point when professional help is key in terms of getting your loved one to hospital and the antipsychotic medication they need to redress the balance of the brain's neurotransmitter imbalance. From my experiences, working with professionals, at the time of a crisis through to discharge, is intrinsic to the well-being and recovery of the service user.

How would a member of the public react if a psychotic episode happens to your loved one when out on their own, for example perhaps in a town centre? How do you help someone suffering from a loss of reality? What would you do in a crisis? Do you know how and where to get help? What would you do in a crisis?

- Call for an ambulance if necessary.
- Check to see if the person has a phone on them for identity. Some carers have (ICE), 'in case of emergency', on their phone, this may well be the case with the service user too. Their main carer's name and number may be on the phone too.
- Would you stop to help, or would you just pass him by whilst yelling rude and mocking remarks? (It has been known.)

**There's a Frog in the Basement: Against the Rules** I was in the throes of doing some paperwork at home, whilst Jay was with his support worker, when the phone rang.

"Hello, Jay."

"Mum?"

"Yes, hello love. Are you alright?"

"No, not really."

"Why, what's wrong? Have you still got someone with you?"

"No, they've gone now."

"What! At this time? That's early. Why?"

"Because she came in and said that it would be just a quick tidy up today, as she has to leave early."

"Well, no one's informed me about her leaving early. Anyway, they can't just please themselves when they leave, they are contracted to work four hours. If you were not feeling too well and you asked them to leave early then that is a different matter. Did you ask them to leave early?"

"No, Mum."

"Are you okay?"

"Yes, but I need to go to the shops."

"Okay, I'll come up, but first I am going to ring the support agency." I immediately rang them and told them what had happened. They did not know the support worker had gone early either.

The agency were shocked to hear what had happened and said exactly the same as I'd said, that care support workers could not just please themselves what time they left, nor could they just decide how little they would do in terms of helping the service user.

They have a contract and service users have a care plan, both of which have to be followed. The manager was extremely apologetic, and said she would speak to the person concerned, and true to her word it was quickly sorted out, however, the person concerned never came back to support Jay.

**What Now?:** A gentleman I know really well, his name is Keith, cares for his wife Lorna who has many different physical and mental health difficulties.

"The level of care I give my wife has risen," he told me. "It's not just basic care, it is now nursing care, and I desperately need medical resources such as syringes, dressings and pads, I can't get hold of the district nurse to bring us some more."

Keith continued, "The prescription for these items was sent by email to the pharmacy, however, it went to the wrong pharmacy. The prescription was sent again, but this time to two different pharmacies. When I rang them, they said they did not have the prescription. A bit later, I rang again. Yes, we have it in they said, but on checking they discovered they did not have the script in. The staff said 'Oh sorry. No it isn't,' and then, 'Sorry, it's actually still on the van. It will be here later.

"But it wasn't still on the van," said Keith. Janet, their support worker, goes back to the pharmacy later to see if it has arrived and to collect it, but it is still not there. When she went back a couple of hours later, as requested by the pharmacist, Janet finally gets the much-needed resources for Keith.

What should be a simple procedure turns out to be a massive barrier in terms of mixed messages, chasing people up with telephone calls and wasted journeys to the chemists.

Keith said to Janet, "I am 77 now, when are professionals going to start understanding the complexities of caring and make a carer's life easier?"

---

## Working Between and Across Government Department

### Legal Roles and Finances

"Being a legal appointee means nothing to us"

### Lived Experience 6 (Approx. 1988-1989)

For working age adults who have learning difficulties, mental health problems, and any other condition that impairs the reasoning, rationality and practical organisation skills, money management can be a great worry to many of them and their carers. Carers are not only managing their own finances, but also the finances of the person we care for. For some service users with difficulties, money in some cases is just an article of trade in order to purchase bits and bobs, paraphernalia or valuables without realising just how much they are spending.

Jay spent most of his money on CDs, hundreds of them, but I must admit he did have good taste in music, and not just one specific genre, it ranged from club anthems, rock, Dire Straits, Pink Floyd, pop, rap and all the songs from the 60s through to the 90s. Numerous carers I have spoken to say their loved one is the same, with money going on whatever they think is relevant to them, at the time, whether they need it or not.

Jay's passion is music, just as fashion is to another, and very often these items take priority as opposed to bills that have to be paid and food purchased to live on. It is not a deliberate act, more a sin of omission than commission, albeit it is an aspect that some service users need help and support with.

The practicalities and consequences of obtaining a loan/s, in which they have no concept of the interest rates charged or paying back the loan, can as we know create a massive problem when trying to sort it out for them.

There must be some way I can help my son budget to ensure that all the priorities such as rent, food and bills are met, with anything left over as personal spending money. So I decided that, in the first instance, to ring the DHSS to find out if there was any help available on this subject.

When I had fully explained the whole situation, they told me I could become his legal appointee. I discussed this with Jay, and he agreed it would be a good idea. It would mean, I explained to him, that in order for me to become his legal appointee, a representative would have to visit us both, from the DHSS's part, to ensure that Jay understood what having a legal appointee meant and if he agreed to it. Jay's consent on its own, for me to deal with the finances on his behalf, was not sufficient enough to help him when dealing with banks, and other organisations, where money was concerned, the legal aspect had to be more authentic.

I was so fed up of trying to set up direct debits to pay monthly bills, to budget and make calls on his behalf, and strive to get problems or queries sorted out without being grilled, quizzed and interrogated every time I contacted an organisation. Thinking that becoming a legal appointee was going to be a godsend, the answer to all the financial worries about managing Jay's budget and housekeeping, in addition to having a joint account into which his benefits would be paid, we hoped it would give me and Jay peace of mind. How wrong I was.

Authorisation was approved for me to be his legal appointee, and all went well for a while. I set up two joint accounts, in both our names, a current account and a savings account, with Jay's benefit being paid into the current account. Bills were now paid on time, food was in the cupboard, there was a personal allowance for Jay and, wherever possible, a few pounds were put into the savings.

One day, several months later, Jay asked me if we could go to the bank for some of his money. I said yes of course we could. (This was before I banked online.) I never thought to ask him, at that point, how much he was wanting. I assumed, wrongly, he would only want about £30, so I was shocked when, once we were in the bank, he said he wanted all of his savings, all £600, which had taken absolutely ages to save.

It was Jay's money after all, and I was only the caretaker of it, but I did explain to Jay that it was not a good idea to just draw out all of his savings only for it to be frittered away, and suggested he just have a couple of hundred instead.

"It takes months to save and it's gone in a day," I said. I had a feeling this would make no difference. I explained to the cashier that I was Jay's legal appointee.

I advised Jay again about taking just a small amount from his savings, as once it had gone, it's gone, and it takes a long time to save up again. Jay became agitated and started to get angry with me; his focus was on having all his savings there and then. I had no idea what he wanted to buy with it. The bank was full of people at the time, and I could feel the lump in my throat getting bigger.

Knowing this was a difficult situation and that I was upset, the cashier left me gobsmacked when she said, "Jay can withdraw all his money."

I reminded her that this was a joint account and surely that meant that we both had to sign for a withdrawal.

"No," she replied. "He can withdraw it himself."

"But I am his legal appointee for this very reason."

"Being a legal appointee means nothing to us. He can have his money."

"But I have a document," I said, waving it in front of her. "I have this document from the DHSS which proves I am his legal appointee."

What she said to me next just totally obliterated any hopes I had of helping Jay with his money.

The member of staff said, "Legal appointees are not officially recognised by banks, so your son can withdraw his money."

When I applied to be a legal appointee for my son with the DHSS, the fact that banks do not recognise this role and responsibility was never mentioned to me when a representative came to see us. All my efforts to try and get something put in place to help Jay with his money, yet again, amounted to another barrier. Well, I can tell you that this barrier was just too much and, at this point, the lump in my throat instantly erupted followed by a myriad of tears. Savings which had taken years to accumulate, which were to be a little nest egg for his future, were gone in a few moments.

I could barely speak, as the cashier handed Jay all his £600 of savings. Naïvely, Jay did not think anything was wrong.

"Thanks, Mum. I'm going to the shops, Mum. Love you lots."

"Love you too, Jay. Take care, look after your money, and do not spend it all," I shouted after him. Guess what? He did.

Every penny was spent, in addition to clinching himself a deal with credit card to boot and racking up a debit of over a £1,000, which he could not pay back. The debt ended up in the hands of a debt-collecting company, which took a very long time to pay off.

I phoned the DHSS to tell them about this incident, and particularly, what the bank had said, that being a legal appointee was not recognised by banks only recognised by the DHSS themselves.

The DHSS said, "Yes, that is true."

"Well why didn't you tell me that before? You knew I needed to manage Jay's money at the bank, I told you this when the DHSS came to see us." I was met with silence.

> **Personal Reflection**: To this day, I still cannot believe this unnecessary incident happened, and I still feel that the cashier made a big mistake that day. The DHSS did not listen to what was really needed in order for the carer to act in their loved one's best interest, the two organisations that should be working together, in order to help carers and service users, in this case were not. I was left feeling devastated and confused.
>
> - Why was Jay allowed to walk out of the bank with all his savings when we had a joint account?
> - Why wasn't I given all the facts relating to being a legal appointee?
> - Why are credit cards given to people with the mental health problems without first finding out if they can pay it back?
> - Why don't the debt collection agencies check to see if the client has any medical problems/benefits/carers?
> - Frightened of the consequences
> - Humiliated in the bank
> - No understanding of how the carer is feeling
> - Incorrect information
> - Why have joint accounts?
> - Lack of information
> - Shocked to learn that a legal appointeeship was meaningless in this instance

**There's a Frog in the Basement: Grace's World** My husband and I were visiting my dad in the cardio ward where my dad was an inpatient; he also suffered with severe Alzheimer's and had a cancerous tumour on his leg. We were told that he was due to go down for an echocardiogram, thus going on to explain that this creates pictures of the heart on its size and shape and checks on how well the chambers and valves are working. Despite my father's illnesses, he always had a twinkle in his eye, a tender mischievous smile on his face, although he did not suffer fools gladly, and his approach to life was optimistic and positive.

The porter arrived to take Dad for his test, and we followed. I have been with my dad for every single doctor's and hospital appointment, and for tests he has needed, since he became ill, and due to his Alzheimer's, I have always gone into the consulting and test room with him in case he gets agitated and needs reassurance, and of course to answer any questions they ask.

After the porter had found an appropriate place to site the wheelchair, my husband and I sat down next to Dad on the chairs in the waiting room.

Surprisingly, the waiting room was not very busy, and the other patients there seemed to be being seen and coming out quite quickly. Dad kept asking where we were, and why we were at the hospital. He had a series of questions that he always asked and would repeat these questions every few seconds. He was always satisfied with our answers, even though he never remembered them, so the whole sequence would begin again.

The door opposite opened, and a lady came out with notes in her hand and called my dad's name.

I immediately stood up and got hold of the wheelchair to take Dad into the room, when the lady doing the test said, in a very abrupt manner, "You can't come in."

Before I had had chance to say anything, she took the wheelchair and wheeled him straight into the room letting the door slam behind her.

I turned to my husband and said angrily, "What was that all about? I always go in with my dad in case I have to explain, or give information to either of them. Dad needs me to explain what he is there for and what they are doing, in a way that he understands, because he can't always hear or understand what some professionals say because they mumble or speak too softly, and what about when the professional needs information? My dad does not remember whether he has even eaten anything let alone anything else." My husband totally agreed with me.

I sat back down in the waiting room feeling, to put it mildly, a bit irritated, when another porter entered the waiting room wheeling a trolley bed, and planted it at the side of the end chair that I was sat on.

The waiting room now only had a couple of patients there, so it was very quiet, apart from the hum of a fan. I casually glanced at the elderly lady on the trolley bed, who I have named Grace, who was talking to herself, at the same time as trying to get something out of her bag. Suddenly, her bag slipped from her grasp and fell on to the floor. I picked it up straight away, as it had fallen to my side of the chair. I stood up and gave her the bag back. She thanked me, and I asked if she was alright. She said something, but I could not quite make it out. I smiled at Grace and sat back down again.

The next moment, Grace was grappling with the bedspread covering her, trying to fling it aside, at the same time as making a move to get out of the bed. I stood up again and asked if she was alright, she didn't answer.

I said, "Please don't try and get out bed, love, or you may fall and hurt yourself."

I looked up to see if there were any nurses around to assist. Neither my husband nor I could see anyone, the place was empty.

A few seconds later, a porter arrived, this time without any trolley or persons. I told him about Grace trying to get out of bed and, with a spring in his step, he went to her aid.

In a jovial voice he said, "Now, love, what are you doing? Let's have you back in bed before you fall." He straightened the bedspread and tucked her in. "How's that then, are you comfortable now, love?"

"Yes, thank you," Grace replied.

My husband was engrossed in a newspaper. The waiting room was empty now apart from us and Grace on the trolley. I could hear very faint, muffled voices coming from somewhere in the hospital corridor.

I sat back in my chair, closed my eyes and relaxed in the silence, only for a few seconds, when I heard Grace say, "Hello, dear, it's good of you to call."

I looked around, wondering who she was talking to.

"No, I'm not. Olive is with me." I realised, on looking at Grace again, that her left hand was in the same position one would use when holding a telephone. With her head and hand turned to her left ear, she continued the conversation. "Olive is just making a cup of tea." Head back to the right. "It's in the green cupboard on the top shelf, dear." Head back to the left. "It's good to hear you, dear." Head back to the right. "Have you found the sugar?" Head back to the left. "Are you alright, dear?" She listened.

Grace was painting a picture in my imagination of her resting in her sitting room, her kitchen, which she could see from where she was sat, which comprised of green wall cupboards, and Olive, perhaps a good friend looking for the sugar and not finding it because there wasn't any left, or Grace had put it somewhere else.

"Oh, that is good to hear." Head back to the right. "It's my son William, he's a doctor." Head back to the left. "Yes alright, I will, hope to see you soon. Goodbye then, dear. I'll come and help you now, Olive."

Grace's hand flopped on to the bedcover, and she closed her eyes. *Wow*, I thought, and sat in silence watching her doze off. I was jolted out of my reverie when the door opposite opened and the abrupt, stout nurse pushed my dad back towards us.

"That's it, all done." It takes approximately twenty minutes to do an echo test, yet in that time, I felt I had been transported into Grace's world for far longer than that and what a privilege it was.

**What Now?:** I checked the landline when I arrived home later that evening. A labour-saving, unmanned message awaited. Then a calm, clear, absolutely toneless, flat and impersonal automated voice spoke to me.

"You have an appointment on the 26th April at 10 a.m. please press 1 to accept or 2 to change the appointment."

Talking to myself again, "Oh, for goodness' sake! How can I do that when I don't who the appointment is for? It could possibly be an appointment for my father, who also has prostate problems, or it could be for me, on the other hand it could also be for my mother or Jay."

The irritating monotone voice did not inform me who the appointment was for, nor which hospital it was at and, considering I care for three family members and myself, all of whom have hospital appointments, the bearer of such notices was not forthcoming with any clues and was no help at all.

I had to press a key to confirm it was me answering the phone. Still talking to myself, irritable and frustrated, I said, "Yes it is me answering the phone, but it is not me who needs the appointment."

"Press 1 to accept the appointment."

More irritable and frustrated, I snapped, "How can I accept the appointment when I do not know who it is for?"

"Press 2 to change the appointment."

Now completely exasperated, I muttered, "Even if I wanted to, how can I change the appointment when I do not know who it is for in the first place?" This was not an option.

Is it possible, I ask myself, to make these messages simpler to respond to? Why can't they give us more options, at the least, to let them know I have tried to get through?

"I am carer with three people to look after, just tell me who the flaming appointment is for, or tell me which hospital it is at the start of the message, and leave me a contact number so I can get back to you."

There is an assumption that it is going to be the patient for whom the appointment is for, answering the phone, yet when a carer is caring for more than one person, in situations like these, how am I supposed to respond? How can we make these systems more user-friendly for carers?

---

**Working Between and Across Government Departments**

**Direct Payments**

**What are the consequences when changes are made?**

**Lived Experience 7**

What are the consequences to the service user and carer when policies change? The manager explained to me that he had not realised that this reshape would have such a drastic effect on the support and care of the service user (Approx. 2006).

The main purpose of direct payments, when it was first introduced, was to empower service users, to give them control over their own social needs and care provision, with the aim of being able to achieve a certain amount of independence, in addition to making their own choices which are vitally important in an individual's life.

This was a remittance that could be used to pay for recreational and social activities, such as going out with a friend or key worker to the cinema, enjoying a sandwich and a beverage in a café, swimming, bowling or whatever other interest one has, a remittance that could be used to embark on educational courses, or resources to use at home, and in college, such as a laptop. A payment, which worked so well in providing a service user with choices that would have once enhanced their lives and that now had been revoked.

Jay had been receiving direct payments for several years, which I managed on his behalf. We chose to pay an agency for a support worker for 10 hours a week, spaced out over two and half days. Direct payments also gave him the opportunity to go on a music course learning about decks and DJs. The location of the venue meant that Jay needed to get a taxi there and back, as it was too far to travel by bus due to the distance, his lack of confidence and anxiety when in the hustle and bustle of a busy town that he does not know, in addition to travelling on his own, especially during winter days and dark nights.

Extremely enthusiastic and enjoying the course, Jay never missed a week, and he received a certificate at the end of the course. Direct payments also allowed Jay to attend the hospital gym, again using a taxi to get there and back. His care package from the agency was in two parts, the first one to help with domestic chores and making a meal etc. and the second part for social interaction, and it worked successfully.

Several years later, due to cutbacks and changes in direct payments, a review was held with the social worker, Jay and me. We discovered that mileage was not going to be allowed any more, therefore, in terms of social interaction, Jay would not be able to go to the following:

- Gym
- Play pool
- Enjoy a ride out in the car with his care worker
- Visit a home and gardens for a walk
- Go to a shopping mall or town centre

"He can use the bus," she said.

Yes, of course, there is always the bus. Well, actually there isn't, because by the time they get a bus and travel into the town, have a quick coffee, there is no time to do anything else, because the support worker has to get back in time for the end of her shift, and she may also have other clients to see after Jay.

When we applied for this payment, and thinking about employing a support agency, I did express the need for transport. A car driver is essential, as sometimes all he would like to do is a have a little ride out somewhere for a change of scenery.

So I sat down and wrote out the places he liked to go, the majority of them being local, for example the supermarket, shopping mall, a ride out and the snooker centre. Along with each of these trips, I included how many miles it was for each one there and back, and consequently gave a total mileage and its costs, with the final total being very little. This change in direct payments ruled out all social interaction, leaving the monies to pay only for invoices from the agency.

At the latter end of the social worker's review and her explanation on the changes to this payment, we both disagreed with the review and refused to sign the form. Jay said, at the time, that the support workers would be coming in to virtually babysit him and, as a thirty-six-year-old young man, he did not want or need babysitting. I fully agreed with him and added that this change would not give him the opportunity to do the small and valued tasks and activities in life that were important to his well-being, the things he enjoyed and benefited from. The social worker said she would go back to the office, contact the manager of direct payments and get back to us.

Consequently, I wrote a letter of complaint, following the

complaints procedure, which outlined the effects these changes would have on Jay and, not only that, for me as his carer as well, because those hours that Jay is with his key worker allow me to have a few hours' respite.

The reply I received was not satisfactory, so I wrote another letter in response. Following this, I had a phone call from the manager of the direct payments department to which he suggested a meeting. I said I would welcome a meeting. This took place several weeks later at my home. The manager was very pleasant, understanding and listened and, after a long discussion, he explained that he had not realised that this change would have such a drastic effect on Jay's support and care, and that he was going to reinstate the direct payment change with immediate effect, therefore the mileage for the support agency was granted, taxi fares were not. Respite allowance was allowed.

- I have tried to claim carer's allowance which would have been of some help, but I was told that if I did claim it, whatever I got, that same amount would be deducted from Jay's benefit, therefore I have never had any form of carers allowance in forty years.

- Even if one does claim the allowance, it is taken away as soon as a person becomes of pensionable age.

- I am an unpaid carer, sometimes working 30 plus hours, along with being on call every night. A support agency gets paid and they pay their care workers, but the law and policies state that the main unpaid family carer is not allowed to be paid out of direct payments by the service user. So I do not receive any payment to help me, and I am doing more hours than the paid care workers.

- Other carers may have different experiences, yet there are still mixed messages as to what direct payments can be used for.

- According to the Rethink Mental Illness fact sheet, it states the different things one can spend direct payments on: this information is correct at the time of writing. These include taxis, help with shopping or budgeting, educational classes, respite and going to the gym. It also states that one can use direct payments to pay a relative to care for the service user as long as the carer does not live with them.

- Are direct payments working for those who need it?

From my experience, the support agency is very good, and if there are any problems they address the issues and find a solution. They are approachable and friendly and, more importantly, always have Jay's best interests as top priority. The manager works with both of us on the care support plan and reviews, and recognises the work the carer undertakes and how important this is to the service user.

---

**Personal Reflection:** I felt upset at the way the review was handled, in terms of both me and my son being put through unnecessary stress and anxiety. The social worker was only doing her job, yet from the onset of the review it seemed as though the decision to cut vital provision had already been made and it was just a matter of signing the form.

---

Decisions that affect a person's life should be discussed with the service user and carer, and in our case, this did not happen until I complained. Carers are still getting mixed messages about direct payments.

Writing official complaints can be so time-consuming, in order to right an injustice, but it has to be done. Carers are always aware of their loved one's feelings and try to keep these emotions stable with reassurance that issues will be sorted out when things go wrong, even though I am spitting feathers.

If they are on a course, maybe voluntary work in some cases, or learning a new activity, transport to the venue is necessary for the following reasons:

- Lack of confidence about going to the venue on their own for the first time
- Anxiety on cold, dark winter nights
- Catching a bus
- Not sure about directions
- Anxious about meeting new people
- Not knowing what to expect when they get there
- Eliminates the service user's and carer's anxiety

At least when a taxi picks them up, and brings them home, and there is someone to welcome them when they get to their destination, both carer and service user have peace of mind to know that their activity has gone well, it has been enjoyed, the people there were friendly, welcoming and helpful, and everything has worked out alright.

**There's a Frog in the Basement: What a Palaver** I collect my son's daily medication and have been doing for many years now. Four tablets a day, which counteracts the side effects of an injection he has every week. Because my son is prone to overdosing, these tablets are given daily.

One Monday morning, I went along to collect the meds, only to be told that the daily medication would no longer be given as a daily medication, but I would have to collect them weekly.

Recently the pharmacy had been taken over by another company, and I was told that they were not allowed to distribute daily meds, and that all the years they had been doing this was down to their goodwill.

I questioned and discussed this matter with the pharmacist, trying to find a solution that would work for us all. Unfortunately, the staff did not think the same way, even when I suggested that, surely, we should all be working together to look at options and come up with an appropriate solution. I was met with silence.

At that time, the pharmacist said they would continue to give the daily meds until the time it changed. I asked when this change was to take place, they said in a week's time. I went to collect the daily meds on Tuesday and was given a week's supply.

I said, "I thought this wasn't changing until next week?"

"No. It's changed now."

The following Monday, I went back again for that week's supply, but I was given just one day's meds.

"I thought it was weekly?"

"Well," they replied, "they have not sent enough, so it's just one day today, and we should have the rest in tomorrow."

The day after, there were only two days tablets and, by this time, I was feeling more than exasperated.

I said, "I would like a full week's supply by the end of this afternoon when I come back at 5 p.m. and, in addition to that, you can take my son off the list at this pharmacy, as I am going to go to another one."

When I went back the meds were ready.

In the meantime, I registered with another pharmacy. All went well for a couple of weeks, until the same thing happened again. They put it on a weekly prescription. Not long after that, it was changed to monthly. The pharmacist, however, did say to me that as long as I was monitoring the medication, monthly should be fine and it saved me coming in every week.

"Okay," I said, "I'll see how it goes."

Again I raise these questions:
- Is there a reason that consultants, GPs and pharmacists cannot work together?
- When I asked my son's consultant about daily meds being prescribed, he said he would write to the doctor, but he could not demand the GP did it that way.

He added that, although Jay was prone to overdosing, the medication he was on would not harm him if he took more than he was supposed to. This problem was not solved in a day; it took a couple of weeks. To date, I now ring for Jay's script and collect it, which is for 28 days. This was a frog in the basement that needed absolute priority. At times, throughout the conversation with the pharmacy, I felt patronised by staff who acted in a supercilious manner. I had discussed this issue with them several years earlier, and I was given the following reasons as to why they could not give medication on a daily basis:

- It was because of time, money and GPs.
- GPs did not write daily prescriptions, it cost them too much.
- Because the pharmacist had to pay for the bottle that the tablets would go in.
- Because they did not get paid to transfer the tablets into individual bottles or the time to do this.
- How do service users manage when they have no carer, guardian or family to monitor medication?

## Dual Diagnoses/Over-the-Counter Medication

The service user may not intentionally want to harm themselves but, at the same time, is looking for a coping mechanism and/or it could be a psychological dependency in which the service user truly believes it will help them. The following might be some of the service user's 'supports' that they think will help them:

- Over-the-counter tablets to aid sleep taking more than the prescribed dosage
- Taking more than a prescribed dosage of medication
- Drugs
- Alcohol

Sometimes, like other issues with organisations, it seems to me that carers have to fit in with the needs of the company instead of the other way round.

Although still being able to ring the GP's surgery for appointments, more recently it seems that booking online is the optimum; however, the problem here for me as a carer, is that I can only book an appointment for myself online, but not for Jay, I have to ring to make one for him.

It is the same with repeat prescriptions. When the pharmacy told me that ordering online for prescriptions was going to be more favourable, as opposed to telephone orders, I discovered that I could do this for my script but not for Jay, simply because online is not set up for the carer to use for the service user to enable them to request a repeat script or appointment.

**What Now?:** Many years ago, my parents took out a funeral plan and paid for it all so that the cost did not fall to me and my sister. My parents' wishes on how they wanted their own funerals to be carried out were all included in the plan. Some years later, my mother had a stroke and my father became progressively worse with severe Alzheimer's. From that moment on, life changed for me and my family.

As lasting power of attorney, I got on with the paperwork that had to be done in terms of letting organisations, such as utilities, insurance etc., know that my parents had now moved back to the area where I lived, and where my parents had lived before retirement. However, they were now both in care homes.

I contacted the funeral directors, where my parents' funeral plan had originally been set up, in order to transfer the details and monies paid to another funeral directors in my area; they told me this was not a problem. *Great, I thought, for once this will be a simple hitch to sort out.* They proceeded to give me a number to ring where it could be dealt with. So I did.

However, there were only two other funeral directors listed on this prearranged payment plan, and neither of them were in my area, which meant I could not use them when the time came, as they were miles away. Consequently, this is how the conversation went:

"Please could you tell me the name of the funeral directors that are part of this funeral plan, and where they are located in my area."

"Two," she said.

"Right, okay, and where are they located?" The first one she mentioned, I estimated was at least fifteen miles from where I lived and the other even further than that. "That's no good," I said, "I need local ones. When the time comes to implement this plan and my parents' wishes, I do not want to be travelling far." I thought this was going to be easy, it was too good to be true.

The lady on the other end of the phone said she couldn't help because she was located at a call centre down south and did not know the areas that these two funeral directors she spoke of were. She had no idea where Leeds was, the area I was ringing from. She said herself that she did not have any geographical knowledge about distances.

"Are there any others?" I asked.

"No, sorry, just those two that are in the plan, but we are hoping to expand with many others in the future."

"In that case then, may I have a refund so I can contact a funeral director in my locality?"

"Yes, we can do that." Why didn't she give me this option in the first place?

With all the evidence she needed of the previous plans and payment, the transaction to refund the monies was made into my parents' account. I discussed all this with my mother, and she then made the decisions for herself and my dad on which funeral director she wanted to use.

After discussions with the new funeral directors, everything was set in place again. I typed up my parents' wishes on all aspects of the funerals they wanted. This was another, fundamental but not pleasant job; however, with copies in place at the care home and the funeral directors, the task was completed.

The previous funeral plans covered the cost of both parents' funerals, but at the time this had to be changed to another area the cost of funerals had risen. I discovered that the monies previously paid would now only cover some of the cost of one funeral; therefore, we took a new plan out in which we could make monthly payments to make up the full cost of one funeral. This means that whichever parents' demise is first, the monies will cover that funeral. As for the second parent's funeral costs, well, we will have to deal with that when the time comes.

**Local Authority**

**Talks about Finances and Care Homes**

**Lived Experience 8**

**Bedheads and Bath Boards**

> *Why, as elderly as I am, do I struggle with a life askew*
> *Looking for a new world to pursue*
> *After all the many years we have lived through*
> *Yet I want to proclaim now, before our visit ends once more*
> *The words you whisper to me*
> *Over numerous cups of tea*
> *Is that I am growing old gracefully*
> *And know that I am accepting this new existence with glee*
> *Especially when you tell me that there's something truly*
> *fantabulous in me*

One of the projects I participated in, as a carer at Leeds University, was called Spotlight: Care Home Research, Promoting relevant evidence – base for care homes. I attended the conference and consequently wrote a reflection of the day:

**University of Leeds – Annie's reflection of the School of Healthcare Education and Debate [SHED] on Care Homes**

School of Healthcare Education and Debate (SHED) talk 12th February 2019.

Enhancing, maintaining and promoting quality in long-term care is a key focus for everyone who lives in, has a loved one in, or works in a care home, as well as for providers and commissioners of care homes, scientists or researchers. Research is vitally important within any organisation, especially when all professionals, carers and service users work together in partnership with researchers to undertake studies that will make a difference to people living or working in care homes.

The School of Healthcare (University of Leeds) has a carer and service user group to support research and education in the school; the group is inclusive and welcoming. As a member of this group, I consider it a privilege to have been invited to contribute as a carer to the Study Steering Committee for a national-funded study to understand the relationship between staffing and quality in care homes.

Below is one of the presentations at a recent School of Healthcare Education and Debate (SHED) event at the university, in order to share research recently completed or being undertaken in partnership with care homes. I have detailed the broad range of research presented at this event which was inspiring; researchers working with people who live and work in care homes to address questions that will make a difference for them. As a carer, I wanted to reflect on this event and what it means for me.

Research topics covered at the SHED event

- Nurturing innovation to enhance care
- Quality and continuity of medication management when people living with dementia move between the care home and hospital setting
- Identifying clinical uncertainties for care homes
- Caring for residents living with frailty
- Proactive healthcare for older people in care homes
- Sexual intimacy and relationship needs in care homes
- Sustaining implementation of new approaches in care homes
- Research enhancing physical activity in care homes
- Relationships between care home staffing and quality of care
- Levels and patterns of physical activity and sedentary behaviour
- Organising general practice for care homes
- Posture and mobility training for care staff versus usual care in care homes
- Innovations to enhance health in care homes

I was a carer of forty plus years for my son and eight plus years for my parents at the particular time of the event. I soon realised that care for a working age adult in their own home, along with caring for elderly parents in a care home, is demanding: the needs of my son and parents are wide-ranging and disparate in terms of certain needs. There have been challenges for sure, but I have also learnt a lot. My father lived in four different care homes, and my mother two. Having been in separate care homes since going into care, due to different physical and mental health conditions, my mother eventually moved to the same one as her husband wanting to be with him through his illness and end of life. My experience of visiting them regularly and working with care home staff to promote quality of care and life for my parents has taught me a great deal about care homes, despite having worked in care homes myself. I have witnessed both good and poor practice in the various homes that I have visited. So what mattered to me? Professionals on Care Home Research covered the following keynote areas:

Nurturing innovation identifying clinical uncertainties:

- Proactive healthcare of older people in care homes
- Sustaining implementation of new approaches in care homes
- Relationships between care home staffing and quality of care
- Organising general practice for care homes
- Innovations to enhance health in care homes
- Quality and continuity of medication management: when people who are living with dementia move between the care home and hospital setting

There is an enormous responsibility that comes with being a carer for elderly parents: maintaining dignity and promoting quality of life and access to services and care are non-negotiable priorities as a carer. Knowing how to deal with community services when your relative is in a care home can feel daunting: yet you are trying to ensure they have basic healthcare needs met, for example hearing, sight, and dental health needs or continence care. Carers have to learn how systems work and how to access services: you are not given a handbook on procedures or processes to follow when having to deal with the inevitable health problems associated with ageing.

How do I get my dad another set of dentures when he placed his on his half-finished dinner plate that was emptied down the garbage chute when staff cleared away? He had eaten most of his meal. I just wonder why the staff did not spot his pair of pearly whites staring at them. Was it because they were placed strategically under the last spoonful of the tasty, stringy cabbage that he decided he did not want after chewing it and spitting it out?

Whose job is it to inform us of any changes in advance? I only discovered, by chance, that when my mother needed new batteries for her hearing aids that it is now a white card one needs when collecting batteries, instead of a yellow card. As a carer looking after every single aspect of a person's life, you have to remain observant, mindful and prudent, and be prepared for whatever barriers and injustices that comes before you. Engagement and discussion between staff and relatives about these small, but important, matters is crucial and will enhance care for both the resident and the carer.

Research of the calibre that I listened to at this event has been outstanding in terms of the questions being asked, ways of working and findings of relevance. The language used at the event instilled a feeling of hope for me in appreciating the sector and its important role in caring for some of the most vulnerable members of our society. It was great to participate in debate, to raise questions and challenges at this event, to drive this research forward. I congratulate the researchers for engaging a broad audience and for the opportunity to be a partner in your work.

## Background leading up to why my parents had to go into care

When my parents went into different care homes, I was thrown into yet another unknown zone of the caring world. Faced with choosing not just one but two care homes that I could rely on to be respectable, dependable and honourable, care homes that would inspire me with their staff's knowledge, understanding, compassion and dedication to make these homes, my parents' homes, was a frightening choice to have to make when, at times, on the news I had heard that some of them were unethical and corrupt.

I will outline here a little of the background that led up to my parents going into care homes. Ed and Rose enjoyed going to the coast before my sister and I were born, and then lots of day trips there, along with holidays to Wales when we were children. They loved the coastal town so much that they decided to retire there many years ago. Ed and Rose were married in 1950; my father was a highly skilled engineer and my mother an auxiliary nurse.

At the onset of the deterioration of my Dad's memory, the only thing my mother told us was that his memory was not too good, however, over several years, his memory became much worse, and the family had recognised the signs that this was much more than just forgetfulness.

Dad was still driving at the time, and went just about every other day to the local garage to fill the car up with petrol, when it did not need any. In addition to this, he also used the local mechanics to get the car MOT and serviced. The MOT was due and my mother worried about him going to get this done on his own, so we went over to help.

Obviously, the car would have to be left there for the mechanics to do its MOT, so my dad drove his car with me in the passenger seat, and my husband followed in our car, in order to bring us both back after dropping the car at the garage.

It was a cold, rainy day, and my dad was messing about with some switches.

I asked him what he was doing, and he said, "Looking for the windscreen wipers." I found the switch to turn them on and off we went.

It was only a short drive to the garage which included a left turn, as it was a one-way system. I was not too concerned about his driving, at that point, just a little worried, as I could see for myself that he was not sure of the roads or signposts. It was a ten minute journey, which could have had a very different ending when I realised that he was not putting the indicator on to turn left.

With urgency, I shrieked, "Dad, you need to turn left just here," pointing to the road in question.

"I don't," he said calmly.

Shrieking even louder, because we were coming up to the turn quickly, I said, "You do Dad, now, now." He slammed the wheel to the left, veering over the road a little as he did so, but at least we got on to the right road, just at the right time. Now I was convinced that this was not just age-related memory problems, it was something much more serious.

I was devastated to realise that he could possibly have Alzheimer's and that my dad should not be driving. Then wonderful memories flooded into my head when he took me on the back of his motorbike for a ride out when I was a kid, excited and having a great time travelling on the country roads especially the ones with the big dips, where I would say, "Faster, Dad. Faster," down the dip and up again, and another one coming up in seconds. I would whoop and cheer, and Dad would chuckle with that special sparkle in his eyes.

On our arrival at the garage, Daniel told us that Dad had been going in every week, sometimes twice a week, to get the car serviced; Daniel told him that it had just been done and everything was alright. Dad was even getting his wallet out to pay him every time he went in; thank goodness Daniel was a really helpful, honest guy. We talked to Mum about what had happened. Mum then went on to tell us about lots of other incidents that had occurred that she had refrained from telling us about before, because she did not want to worry me and my sister, but it had got to the point where she could not cope any longer on her own. I told her I would get in touch with the GP and take it from there. Dad needed help, and our assumption that it was Alzheimer's he was suffering with was confirmed after tests and brain scans had been completed.

My mother had a stroke in June 2013 and was admitted to their local hospital. Three days later, my dad was sectioned to the local mental health hospital, and a fortnight later, Mum was moved to a stroke rehabilitation centre. Two weeks after this admittance, she went to a convalescent home for six weeks.

In August, after a little over two months of being in hospital, we brought my dad to a care home with nursing in Leeds, and four days later, my mum came to live with me and my husband which we anticipated would be until the end of her life, how wrong we were.

We changed everything around in our home to accommodate Mum, and make her feel at home as much as possible, with a warm and comfortable, downstairs bedroom complete with new bed, and bathroom next to it, she thought it was lovely and was so appreciative.

With caring for my son as well, my days now started at 5 a.m., with Mum already awake, so there was a cuppa first thing to get the day started. Then I helped Mum get up, commode, breakfast, bathed and dressed. Got myself ready, then up to my son's, cleaned, shopped, medication and so on. I arrived back home at 4.30/5 p.m. to get the tea ready and eat tea. Mum would stay up late talking, and as I was usually in bed for 9 p.m., I could hardly keep my eyes open at 11.30 p.m. Then get Mum ready for bed after a bedtime drink, tuck her up and say goodnight, God bless, just like she always did with us as kids after a bedtime story. Usually I got five hours sleep, tops, being on call through the night for my son and mum, the alarm would go off and we'd start all over again. I classed myself as very fortunate, because I know carers whose situations are far more demanding especially when they are dealing with relatives who have far more severe disabilities.

At the latter end of the year, my husband and I, if possible, usually attended the Carers UK conference in London. I asked my mum if she would be okay to go into a care home for respite whilst we were away for one night. She said she would. We found a care home and took her to see it. The staff were welcoming and showed Mum round. She thought the bedrooms were spacious and comfortable, and she met the other residents. On the invitation of the manger, Mum spent a half day with them, then a full day, before going in for respite.

On our return, she said she had really enjoyed being there and chatting with everyone.

One morning, a few days later, when I asked her if she'd slept well, she said no. Mum said she had been thinking all night, long and hard, about the care home and how lovely it was, and that she would like to go and live there. We didn't see that coming. After tea that evening, we stayed up late with her discussing all the pros and cons about what she wanted to do. Her decision however stayed the same.

She was speaking to an aunty one evening on the phone, and I heard her tell her that she was going into a home because if wasn't fair on us, and we had enough to cope with. I told Mum that this was not true, and she could stay with us forever. I tried to convince her that she was not a burden, as she put it, and she was welcome to stay, so there was still time to change her mind. But that did not happen, and that was how Mum came to go into a residential care home.

**Care Homes – What is the difference between them?**

Deciding on a care home, as I discovered, is not as easy as I thought it would be when there are so many aspects to take into consideration, such as the location, services they provide in terms of the health of your loved one, the accommodation and its outside space, and the cost. I have just written a brief description of care homes below, however, you would be as well to write a list of exactly what services and healthcare a home provides, as well as the costs, as each one of our loved ones is different.

Local Authority Residential Care Homes: A residential care home setting provides only personal care, such as washing, dressing and medication. As a rule, most care homes provide activities and entertainment in addition to having a hairdresser and chiropodist, both of which the residents have to pay for. If transport is available, there can be trips out for the afternoon to areas of local interest and/or lunch at a pub. If there are any local performances, such as bands, concerts or choirs that are of interest, these are arranged as well if the resident wishes to go.

Care Homes with Nursing: In addition to the personal care given as above, care homes with nursing employ qualified nurses to deal with other aspects of health that a residential home cannot.

Nursing Home: Is a place for the elderly who are ill and live and receive medical treatment and care.

Private Homes: Some of these are run by companies, individuals and some charities. Private homes are regulated, just like all the others, and are regularly inspected by the Care Quality Commission (CQC). The more luxurious facilities provided by private homes may consist of spas, beauty and barber salons, and treatment rooms for therapeutic services, along with opulent, spacious rooms for quiet rest and relaxation, in addition to several other palatial lounges and bedrooms.

Location of the care home is important so that family can get there easily, particular for the main relatives who liaise with the home on a regular basis and are sometimes called in an emergency, along with considering the travelling expenses.

The majority of homes include an events coordinator, and their role is to organise informal, social programmes that includes activities such as a good singalong, in-house, often inviting musicians and singers to come in and entertain residents, animal therapy, religious services in accordance to the residents own particular faith, in-house radio or CD music to relax to in the lounge, plus various arts and crafts.

Depending on the care home, some branch out into other areas such Alzheimer's, dementia, stroke and other mental health issues. Local authority care homes, and care homes with nursing, use the local GPs and community health services such as matrons, nurses, speech therapists, dieticians, audiologists and optometrist, with some of these being classed at specialist services in private homes. Some homes provide for both residential and nursing care patients.

**Finance and Care Homes**

It is important to be aware of top-up fees if the council are paying towards care. If you choose a care home that is costing more than the council's ceiling for costs per month, you will have to pay top-up fees and these payments are not payable by the resident but by the family.

In terms of cost, with regard to local authority homes, if a resident has £23,250 or more in savings, one is not usually considered for financial help from the local authority, however, if and when these savings reduce, it is the local authority's advice to contact them before savings fall below this amount if you think you are going to need financial assistance. If an individual's savings are £14,250 or less this will be disregarded.

I was told that this amount was ignored in order to pay for funeral costs etc. [Age UK Updated July 7th 2020. *Paying for residential care: capital £23,250 - £14,250*]

A financial assessment, or means test, is carried out by the local authority to determine how much money one has and if the council will pay towards one's care. My family and I had a financial assessment carried out by a financial officer and this was for both of my parents, so it took some time. They look at aspects such as the individual's benefits, investments, savings, income, state pension, private pensions, pension credit, and allow a sum of £24.90 per week for the individual's own person allowance. We had this financial assessment because both of my parents needed to go into different homes because of their individualised health situations.

Applying for a deferred payment means that the local authority would pay part of the monies towards the care home in conjunction with what each parent would pay individually to it. This is basically a loan that has to be paid back when the property is sold on the second person's demise, not the first because, the property is still legally owned by the remaining spouse. On the demise of the last spouse, the property has to be sold and you have a certain amount of time to sell the house before interest accrues.

Although I gradually started to understand how deferred payments worked, I became pretty stressed trying to keep my eye on the ball when it came to keeping track of two lots of payments to two different care homes, two lots of different financial situations in terms of DWP benefits, pension credits, two lots of invoices, payments made to the care home by the local authority, on top of my son's direct payments and invoices from the agency, along with audits and reports for the OPG and direct payments.

I was constantly ringing, or emailing, the financial officer for the abundance of questions I needed to ask, queries I need clarifying and confirmation on all other sorts of different aspects. I am sure a little marker would pop up against the side of my name every time I phoned – *Oh no, it's Annie again.* But if I do not understand any procedures and why they are implemented, I have to ask.

Several years ago, as a carer on the board of the Carers Strategy Implementation Group for Adult Social Services, myself and four other carers had a meeting with the chief executive officer in order to discuss each of the distinct areas that we felt needed clarity and addressing in order to make improvements to all the distinct elements that were, to say the least, bewildering.

The particular issue I had at that time was the financial legislation which I mentioned earlier. Some time after this meeting, it appeared that this bone of contention was not being followed up, so again I reminded them of that first meeting and felt that it needed to be taken further, and I am pleased to say that it was.

The following is a shortened version of the report I wrote for this meeting, when it was arranged between the senior manager and other staff integral to the subject matter for adult social services.

**Report: My report to Adult Social Care Financial Services**

*Are you managing a loved one's finances? We make it simple and undemanding*

**Aims**

This report is written from an unpaid carer's lived experience. Its purpose is to act as a catalyst for discussion, in order to review and develop new and existing, user-friendly communication including systems, policies and procedures for the public. It highlights the many questions carers ask, and should include the expectations of both parties.

Local authorities, including the financial department, have to adhere to government instructions and legislation along with translating this information to carers, service users and financial representatives in a straightforward and uncomplicated way.

This is not an easy task considering the many aspects that are involved in relation to carers who manage their loved one's finances for the following:
- Financial assessments for people who go into care homes
- Financial assessments for people who need support at home
- Financial assessments for people who need care at home with more complex difficulties

Despite each individual's caring situations and circumstances, very often all of the issues we deal with throw up more questions than answers, not always immediately but months on.

Information given, in the early stages of dealing with an unfamiliar scenario, is very harrowing for carers to take in all at once when dealing with extremely stressful, demanding and difficult undertakings.

This then becomes even more problematic when trying to put it into practice, because carers are faced with many questions, and yet more tasks, that we do not know how to answer or how to deal with.

Practically, these situations for carers waste precious time, generate paperwork, and telephone calls, along with the anguish, struggles and headaches each and every barrier brings with it. An issue can leave the carer dealing with several different organisations all at once, who each have a varied take on the same query. Mixed messages and lack of communication for the carer is, again, extremely frustrating, mentally draining and emotionally upsetting.

It is anticipated that by carers and organisations working together, we can eradicate the worry and distress for carers with a solution to these situations by devising and delivering information and procedures in a transparent, undemanding and trouble-free way.

## Objectives

From the above aims and the lived experience, it is hoped the following objectives will be achievable in the near future:
- Discuss local authority guidelines and legislation to ensure that this is being adhered to within a review, and how a user-friendly model within the local authority remit can be adapted.

- Discuss each category with a view to developing a list on how each of the issues can be improved.

- Discuss all aspects and decide what is working and what is not. What we want to achieve, whether it is achievable and, if not, how we can make it achievable with adaptations in terms of information, policies, procedures and systems.

- Ensure clarity and transparency in all forms of communication given to carers.

- To be open and transparent with all information.

- Devise and design user-friendly public information in terms of brochures and booklets.

- Devise and design a carer's package/book that covers all the aspects of everything that a carer needs to know in terms of information, organisations, etc. and one that can be updated on a regular basis.

- Develop engagement and co-production with DWP, care homes, social services, local authorities and the finance sector. In the past, I have organised events with staff from the mental health services, putting into place an event, that carers have asked for, which has incorporated the CEO, psychiatrists, director of nursing, and many other medical and non-medical, senior staff in mental health.

These events give carers and service users an opportunity to ask questions of the right professional. Do you think we will ever see any similar events in the future with other corporate organisations, where carers can ask professionals in banks, DWP and Job Centres the questions we would like to ask without trailing from place to place and making numerous phone calls?

Some professionals are invited into carers' events, such as solicitors, where the professionals speak about a specific topic, such as lasting power of attorney, or wills, which gives the carers chance to ask questions and gain new and updated information, which is brilliant. The other advantage is that all carers present learn something from all the questions and answers on the day.

## Financial Assessment

Because of the varied events leading up to the carer considering a financial assessment for their loved ones, they are probably already, mentally, in an emotional place. Therefore, embarking into another unknown chapter in their lives just accelerates the worry, alongside them having difficulty managing their own finances. Looking after someone else's finances is a massive undertaking, a big responsibility and even more pressure, and I feel that more ongoing support is needed.

Reflecting on this experience, I highlight the strengths and weaknesses of systems and procedures with a view to further consultation on how these issues can be improved. We have a large amount of information to take in all at once and, although we may ask questions at the time of an assessment, it is often later, when we have had a little more time to digest and replay the meeting and what was said, we find that many of the answers only generate more questions, let alone the answers we have forgotten.

There is a great deal of paperwork that the financial officer has to complete with the carer at the start, throughout and beyond the whole process of adult social care services. One of the questions I asked in the early stages was:

- Is there someone I can talk to for ongoing help, support and advice? – You can phone us if you have a problem or question.

I was expecting a financial agreement to include what was expected of both parties, similar to taking out a bank loan, where one receives a contract on exactly how much has to be paid back every month over a certain number of years until the loan is paid off. It is, in fact, the amount of money paid by the resident to the care home for their care that is deducted from the capital of their home when it is sold, and there is a legal contract to sign.

What happens when two parents are on deferred payment on the home they both own, and both have to go into care at the same time? This happened in my case, with my father's demise being first. This means that the property still legally belongs to the remaining spouse. But, because my mother needed full-time care, she had to remain in the care home. However, if the circumstances for my mother meant she had been well enough to have support at home, or only be in the care home for respite, she could have moved back to her own home.

Property can be sold after the first person's demise, even when the remaining spouse is in care, and all monies can be paid back to the local authority, thereby finalising the deferred payment agreement.

In terms of a deferred payment, and the legal contract, a property that is sold on the demise of the remaining spouse states that the property has to be sold within so many days before interest accrues.

It is advisable to keep a check on what the interest fees will be, and if you find this difficult to do seek professional advice. Mistakes can be made, as it was in my case when the local authority charged over £2,000 of interest on the property sale, when in actual fact, no interest at all should have been added due to the fact that he was the first spouse to die and we did not have to sell the property at that time. Interest is only charged on the demise of the second spouse if the property is not sold within the legal amount of time given. Having pointed this error out to the local authority, they checked and apologised for their mistake and refunded the money.

What would have made things a little easier to understand was if the legal contract document was in evidence at the time of the meeting, so we could read through it and have any questions, we had on it, answered.

Although the legal contract is a relatively measured document, I felt it needed to be slightly more comprehensive in terms of detail. I also feel that a user-friendly version should also be considered.

**Deferred Payments** The twelve-week disregard process I found confusing, as one is led to believe that a person does not have to pay anything for the first twelve weeks of the resident being in the care home. However, I was then informed that monies for care have to start being paid immediately. It was also implied that this money would be subtracted and given back when the property is sold. If you are unsure about this process, keep asking questions until you are fully satisfied that you understand the process fully.

**Tick-Box Form** At the end of the financial assessment a tick-box form is completed to confirm what the financial officer has spoken to you about at the meeting. This is a process that is completed very quickly and, given the important information that the carer has already had to take on board, I feel a little more time should be allowed for the carer to process and digest this final part of the assessment.

**Financial Statements of Equity** A property valuation has to be given at the time of a financial assessment, however, it was not mentioned at the beginning of the financial assessment on my parents' behalf that the true equity of the clients' assets cannot be determined until the property is sold, because a final valuation has to be sought, therefore I could not expect to receive any annual statements that showed the balance of what has been paid so far by the resident or what equity is left. I did, on occasions, ring to find out and was given the information, though the answer to all those aspects will only be finalised on the demise of the last spouse when the house is valued and sold.

When I rang the DWP with a query on my parents' behalf, I discovered that they too have the valuation of the property which, on further discussion, was a different valuation to the one I had given to the financial officer, so that was another issue I had to get my head round and resolve.

It is a very confusing and worrying time, and you really have to be astute about how this system works in order to pick up on any anomalies you feel there might be, so below I have listed a few points to consider and keep check of when dealing with your loved ones' financial affairs in these kinds of situations.

- **Personal Allowance** This usually increases when benefits award a cost of living pay increase each year, this is also the time when care fees increase as well. You should be notified about these increases, enabling you to amend, if you have one, a direct payment or standing order at the bank.

- **Notifications** of annual financial assessments, reports and audits, if these are applicable to your situation.

- **Statement of finances**_in terms of the local authority contribution. Be clear about exactly what the local authority are paying towards your loved one's care home fees when on a deferred payment contract.

- **Statement of finances** in terms of client contribution. Be clear about exactly how much your loved one is contributing to their care fees.

- **Overpayments** and underpayments check your invoices and statements carefully from care homes etc.

It took me quite a while to sort out a problem when a care home made a mistake with the finances and had overcharged on monthly payments. They informed me that they had mislaid their remittance advice notes and, as a result, were asking me to pay a substantial amount back which we did not owe. They found their advice notes sixteen months later. Keep a check on payments so you can deal with the discrepancy straight away if you have a query on them.

- Is your loved one a private funder, self-funding or local authority funded? Be clear about what these entail. Check contracts between your local authority and care home, a self-funder does not need a contract. However a resident on local authority funding does.

- Keep an eye on your loved one's benefits i.e. Attendance Allowance, Pension Credits, State Pension, private pensions and other benefits.

- Check the dates that Attendance Allowance starts and stops. My mother's Attendance Allowance stopped and I was not notified about this. This may be brought to your attention at the financial assessment meeting.

Below are the figures I needed most to keep a regular check on:

- Care home contributions that are paid by your loved one.

- Local authority contributions that are paid to the care home.

- Your loved one's State Pension, private pension, Pension Credits, benefits such as Attendance Allowance and any other form of income coming in.

- Your loved one's Personal Allowance. This should also be increased as benefits increase.

Check the figures, keep statements, receipts and invoices and all correspondence because you never know when you may need it. As procedures and polices change, check to see how these may affect things, if at all, and if in any doubt check with the appropriate professionals that can answer your questions.

**Some reminders for your checklist**

- **Information**: Booklets, leaflets, get as much information as you possibly can. If you have any queries after reading the information, jot your questions down and speak to the appropriate person that can answer them.

- **Assessments**: Check what financial and needs assessments have to be made and what they entail for your loved one.

- **Assessments**: If your loved one remains in their own, or your, home for care and support, check what assessments you both need along with the resources and financial help you can apply for.

- **Professionals**: Ensure you know exactly why you need the professional, and what they will be doing to help you, as well as obtaining clarity on the roles and responsibilities of the tasks they are helping and advising you with.

- **Keep a record of:**
  - Interest fees
  - Legal contracts

Also keep records of all your loved one's financial dealings, such as payments, statements and invoices, along with all correspondence, such as letters, notifications on benefits and pensions, Personal Allowance, from all the reputable and established organisations you deal with.

As well as keeping all the files I need for my son, it soon became pretty obvious that I would have to get two extra filing cabinets in my home to accommodate all my parents' files as well.

**Welfare Support**

We worry about how our loved ones will manage, on our demise, in terms of managing their money. That is a thought we carers carry round with us and is talked about in support groups and with professionals. It is a constant potential issue which causes anxiety and concern.

The scenario is this: what happens when a working age adult with mental health problems who has relied on his only parent, the main carer, dies and there are no other relatives to take the place of the carer?

In this particular case, the routine has always been that the service user's benefit is paid into the joint account of the service user and parent, with the parent – main carer – making sure that all bills are paid on a direct debit, monitoring the account, along with transferring fortnightly benefits every week into their personal account.

This is a procedure that works well for them both. But in the event of that parent carer's demise, what happens? The service user would have difficulty in monitoring the direct payments and other accounts that pay for support services etc. due to the services user's condition, whereby they demonstrate a lack of, or poor, organisational, concentration, understanding and memory skills, in addition to the difficulties of reading, retaining and maintaining information, logical thinking and understanding finances. All of these, and more mental and physical disabilities, contribute towards disastrous and devastating effects on the service user when left to their own devices. Unpaid bills and no money left to live on or buy food would just leaving them feeling distraught and exacerbate their mental and physical well-being.

I am led to believe that the local authority's Adult Social Care and Financial Services would step in and take over the necessary and appropriate paying and monitoring of bills. However, in some of the lived experiences I write about, I worry and question the competence and reliability of some of these professionals to carry out this specific job as well I, and thousands of other carers, have been doing and still currently do. I strongly believe that information on exactly what the procedures, policies and services provided in these situations are, should be open, transparent and explained in public information leaflets so we know exactly how to prepare for this event before it happens.

This is the statement I put in my report:

*Do you worry about how your loved one will manage when you die, when there is no one at all to take over the responsibilities of every single aspect of care including finances?*

Maybe I have missed something in my research, but the main source of information on this subject from various establishments seems to be aimed at "What to do when someone you care for dies" when, in actual fact, carers need to know "What can I put in place for my loved one before I die, for the working age adult?".

Much of this information comes from solicitors, where the focus seems to be on elderly people and not on vulnerable, working age adults. Information directs one to the legal aspects of looking after your loved one's finances, such as power of attorney and appointees, etc., in addition to what care the vulnerable person would need who has been left on their own, and again advising one to obtain a needs assessment. Advice and support, it appears, is centred on the physical and practical side of caring for most ages and people with dementia and Alzheimer's.

## Questions I have heard from carers and service users

- *I care for my working age daughter with mental health problems and physical disabilities. My ongoing concerns are what practical, financial and emotional support mechanisms can be put in place by Adult Social Welfare Services to support my daughter when I die?*

- *I have problems with organisational and financial skills. My father is my main carer and helps me on a daily basis to do the cleaning, shopping, washing, ironing, cooking and mange my finances. Are there any provisions we can put in place for someone to help me to do this when my father dies?*

- *I have problems communicating and need help. If I have a problem with queries and sorting out problems with organisations such as utility companies, can social services take this over when my mother dies?*

- *I find it difficult to remember medical appointments to the hospital, GPs, dentist, opticians and when I get there with my brother I cannot remember what they have said to me when I get home, so my brother always reminds me and puts it on the calendar. What provision is there to help me with this problem when my carer dies?*

- *I am not very good with money. Can arrangements be made with social services finances to deduct just my bill money from my benefits for them to pay and monitor my bills every month? Leaving me with the remainder of my benefits to live on.*

- *I get income support which is for my daily living. This goes into an account that my mother looks after and transfers it into my personal account on a daily or two daily bases, sometimes a week's money. When she dies how will I manage to do this?*

- *I do not have a computer and if I had one I do not know how to use it. Where else can I get information on anything I need? I don't want a computer because I would struggle to understand how it works or what to do if I had any problems with it.*

- *I want to stay in my own home which is owned by the local authority. I have a support agency. Would I be able to get extra support from the care agency and my care worker if my mum dies because I have no other family to help me?*

- *I live alone, is there someone I can turn to like a social worker or care support worker for help and support?*

As carers we all need answers to these questions, along with more verbal and written information, on this extremely important issue, because at the moment we are working in the dark with our loved ones, with absolutely no idea of what provisions, if any, are available in the questions asked above and that uncertainty for the future just exacerbates our anxieties even further.

**Conclusion of report:** I thanked everyone concerned, and their colleagues, for inviting me to participate, as a carer, in this forthcoming review of resources and strategies. I trust that by submitting this carers report it will prove to be a useful and productive document for discussion towards a more coherent, transparent, positive and proactive approach for carers when they find themselves in difficult and unknown situations.

Every carer has their own lived experience depicting the different barriers they face every day, and even though I have tried to cover most aspects of the concerns and issues in this document, there are many more to be looked at in terms of carers' different circumstances which again raise questions relevant to their own caring domain.

If changes are considered to reflect a carer and service user's life in terms of making policies, procedures and communication more user-friendly with all the information available, I would suggest that several other carers be involved in future discussions.

**Outcome:** Further to more discussions and telephone calls with Adult Social Services, they produced draft documents on care homes and payments towards non-residential social care services. The latter one: Information about the Adults and Health Charging Policy and how it affects is dated 1st April 2017 to 31st March 2018. Both of these documents were superbly presented in a very clear, precise and user-friendly format.

Let us add to that, a booklet entitled: **Who will help me with my finances when my parent-main carer dies?**

---

**Personal Reflection:** The experiences I have shared above speak for themselves, highlighting the confusion and complexities as well as the frustrations and anxieties that one can, and does, encounter as a carer. They also import and call attention to the fact that more can be done to improve a lot of these areas to take away the sometimes impending feeling of doom, in terms of our prospects and expectations in order to be fully confident that our loved ones will be looked after in all aspects of their lives when that time comes. To complete this section, I leave you with several other experiences that took me to the realms of sheer desperation.

---

### Continuing Care Treatment Assessments (CCT)

The first couple of CCTs my father had showed he did not qualify for this contribution from the NHS. Later, another review was carried out. In attendance at this CCT meeting were two of the senior management team, one being the matron, the other being the manager, the senior nurse conducting the CCT assessment and myself. This assessment again rendered that he did 'not fit the bill' for nursing care.

I didn't think it would, as this was just a usual follow-up from the main CCT carried out six months previously. I was, however, totally stunned and open-mouthed when the manager suddenly declared that my father would have to leave the care home. He said he would have to go to another one to avoid nursing fees accruing any more than they already were.

I said, "How come there are nursing fees when he doesn't even need nursing care? This is the first I have heard about any nursing fees."

I just could not understand this 'out of the blue' demand.

"Why does he have to move? He does not need nursing care, and how can nursing fees possibly accrue when he is not even getting nursing care? You have been sat here whilst this assessment has been taking place and witnessed the senior nurse saying he does not meet the criteria for nursing care, and on top of that moving him with severe Alzheimer's, when he has settled here, will surely be detrimental to his health."

The senior nurse agreed it would be.

There was a moment of silence, until the manager continued with, "He still has to move. We have another home he can go to. It is purely residential, and there are no nursing fees."

"But my father came here as a residential patient with Alzheimer's on the advice of his consultant who said it would be better for Dad to go into a care home with nursing so that when, not if, his condition deteriorates he will not have to be moved to a nursing home. You said that was fine, no problem, so what has happened? Why the sudden change?"

He replied, "To stop nursing fees accruing."

We were just going round in a loop dialogue, despite the fact I tried to discuss the blatantly obvious reason why Dad should not be moved, it was to no avail, and even the senior nurse did not say anything to support me.

This was an unprecedented and unexpected issue, just like many others carers have thrust upon them, we have, in many situations, to really fight for our loved one's well-being. My heart went out to my poor dad who did not know what was going on, oblivious in his own world, and trusted me profusely to always do the right thing for him; literally, his life was in my hands.

Without further discussion from the manager, he got up and left the room. Yes, there was a lump in my throat, but I wasn't going to give them the satisfaction of seeing me cry. I was not going to show any weakness, because I had to stay strong for my dad.

After getting Dad settled to another one of this company's homes, which I had serious doubts about, all seemed to be going well, but that did not last. With my permission, a few weeks later, they moved Dad to another room on a temporary basis and on the condition it would be the same size and layout of the room we had originally selected out of one of three they showed to us.

Because he was transferred to this other room very quickly, I did not see it, but my sister did.

She rang me immediately and said, "Have you seen this room they have moved Dad into? It's appalling," and she was fuming. She went on to say that it was nothing but a broom cupboard with sticky floors along with being dark and dismal, and, without further ado, immediately sent an email to the owners telling of her disgust in that staff could even think about moving a resident to such a demoralising and inadequate room. The problem was resolved instantly.

The last straw was when we found Dad sat in a chair which faced a blank wall, despite the lounge, with other residents in, being behind him. He could not see or speak to anyone from the position they put him in.

After immediately moving him to a more appropriate place in the lounge, our visit was over. I went home and straight away got in touch with the social worker to let them know what had happened. We then had to find another home and, of course, on choosing one, Dad then had to have another needs assessment carried out to ensure that this care home would be able to meet his needs and vice versa.

Did the story end there? I am afraid it did not. In fact, it went on for a further five years, even after my father had died. I started receiving invoices, from the first care home with nursing, for the colossal amount of the best part of £8,000. *What is this for?* I thought, and soon discovered it was for, alleged, outstanding nursing fees. I made numerous phone calls, sent multiple letters, spoke to the accountant, yet still my complaint was ignored and the invoices kept on arriving.

My letters to them stated that my father did not need nursing care, did not receive any nursing care whatsoever, along with the CCT that proved he did not need it. If they were alleging that he did, could they please send me the evidence to corroborate this, in terms of a list describing all the nursing care they purported he'd had, along with the resources they had used, and including the days, dates and times this 'so-called' nursing care had taken place. I did not receive a reply.

This dispute went on for many months, until one day I had a phone call from the accountant, a new accountant, who had no idea of the previous history and had rung to ask why this invoice had not been paid. I had to retell the whole story.

*Here we go again*, I thought. So I told him everything. He said he would look into it, because something was evidently not right. I never heard from him again, but the invoices kept dropping on my doormat. By this time, I was at screaming point. Why was no one listening to me? I had asked for meetings to discuss this further, but my requests were snubbed.

My father's condition worsened, he had undergone an operation on his leg to remove a cancerous tumour and he was deteriorating with Alzheimer's. Because of the nursing care he would need now, and at some point palliative care, the residential care home, without nursing, he was in but catered for people with Alzheimer's, could no longer meet his needs and consequently we now had to move Dad to yet another nursing home.

When he moved into the new home another CCT was carried out and it was, as we expected, that this time he did need nursing care and was awarded nursing care fees. With the upheaval of four removals in total, my dad was disorientated and agitated, and we were all distressed and very tired.

To push our already heightened emotions and fatigue even further were all the meetings we had with the social workers, medical staff and care homes, along with making sure my mum was settled in the care home she was in, and caring for my son, who, in his own way, gave us the love and support we needed at a time when we were feeling totally wiped out. But still the invoices kept arriving.

Not long after moving to a new care home with a confirmed Continuing Care Treatment plan in place, Dad was taken to hospital. After several weeks, the hospital said they were going to do another CCT assessment before my dad was discharged.

A small nurse's station, equipped with computer, was located conveniently next to the six-bedded ward that my dad was on, although he wanted to be walking around all the time. Other patients in there were suffering similar physical and mental medical conditions that my dad demonstrated, in terms of being unsettled, with outbursts of quarrelsome confrontations which he was responding to or instigating, punctuated with minor pockets of inconsequential ructions. It was one of those days, as I sat down with the nurse at the computer to embark on the CCT. I had a copy of the recent CCT, in order to follow what had been stated on it, so I could compare the answers the nurse was putting in to the ones I had.

Every question she filled in made it sound as though my dad had unambiguously morphed back into good health. This was a man who had severe Alzheimer's and a massive, cancerous tumour on his leg. The next question she answered stated that he did not display aggressive behaviour. I asked her how long she had known my dad, and she said since she'd come on duty, so I asked her what time that had been, confirming that she had only known him for the length of her shift that day, to which I politely pointed out that I had known him all my life.

At that point, I saw my dad had wandered down the corridor to the next ward. I was distracted by this as, being prone to falls, he should not have been walking anywhere. Suddenly, the whole department was drowned in a raucous war of words between my dad and another patient. I rushed into see what was going on. My dad was shouting at the other patient because he had accused my dad of being gay.

I then rushed back to the nurse and said, "Before you fill that question in about not displaying aggressiveness, you had better go and see him now," which she did. Finally, when my dad and the other gentleman were settled, I went back to completing the assessment with the nurse.

On comparing the two assessments, every score rated was far lower than the previous one, which meant he was not ill enough to be awarded CCT, when he had already been awarded it and he was on the Gold Standard Framework which again meant that, at some point in the near future, he would need palliative care, yet according to the nurse's account he could quite easily be a stand-in for superman. I said this was not an accurate assessment of my dad's health, and I added that if she printed it to give to me I would tear it up.

Even though I knew the answer before I asked it, I still enquired as to how she could possibly come up with the scores she had done, when she had only known him for a day, and when it was blatantly obvious that he needed nursing care from the recent CCT and seeing him for only a few hours. The nurse did say that she did not know him well. I concluded that the assessment was indeed defective, misleading and, quite honestly, laughable.

At the new care home, staff loved Dad's little jokes, the graceful and pleasing smile he always expressed, along with that sparkle in his eyes when they laughed with him. The tenderness and compassion they showed, as they sat and talked to him, was exceptional. He could not reply, yet the smile on his face told us he was happy. They cared for him as if he was their own father, made him comfortable, cuddled him and demonstrated their skills in caring for Dad, showing the utmost dignity and respect.

Whilst the most calming and soothing music played softly, and steadily, in his warm and peaceful bedroom with subdued lighting, they read his favourite Bible passages and the words to his favourite hymns to him as he entered into the final stages of life. As a family, we did the same, always hoping for one more flicker of recognition from him, to know that we were with him, as we said our goodbyes to a wonderful husband, father, grandfather and friend, as he closed his eyes and went to sleep for the last time.

Still at the beginning of our grieving period, yet another invoice dropped on my doormat, but I could not face dealing with it. They kept on arriving, and it was now two years since my father had died, so when the next one showed itself I was beside myself with anger and frustration. I had had just about as much as I could take from this organisation, and I sat down to write yet another letter.

I could not understand what on earth made the people in this company tick. Their unscrupulousness, and sheer antagonistic methods, and their glaring disregard of what I had been trying to do, over several years, to sort this problem out beggared belief and had now provoked even higher pinnacles of emotion covering me in a suffocating and concentrated veil of fury and outrage.

My letter was not just to them this time, there were multiple letters, as I sent it to a solicitor that I had spoken to some time ago about the case, as the company had threatened to take me to court over non-payment of this invoice. I even wrote back to the company and said words to the effect that implied "Bring it on then, take me to court, at least that way I can see you and state my case".

I told the solicitor everything and took all the letters, invoices and all the documentation I needed in the case file I had been building, including the formal letter and review from the CCT which was sufficient evidence on its own alone to prove he did not need nursing care.

The solicitor said, "If they bring a court case, go, you have a case, you tell them everything you told me, they don't have a leg to stand on, and you don't need a solicitor." I also sent the letter to another eight appropriate companies including the CQC, and three to the CEO, the director and the secretary of the company itself, by recorded delivery.

I would now wait and see what response I would get before

approaching *Watchdog*. I had already had to deal with being accused of fraudulence from a bank (and I dealt with that), so this one, apart from the company's ignorance in dealing with the issue, and absence in all forms of any contact in this so-called nursing fee debt, should be a piece of cake.

I received two responses by phone, and a letter from the CQC. On speaking with the CQC, they asked me to 'hold off' from going public with this matter until they had investigated it. They could not believe that this had been going on for five years. I was quite happy to do what they suggested; at least now someone was taking this matter seriously. Was I relieved not to be alone with this monstrous problem any more, from a company that had me thinking they were all invisible, did not exist at all, or that it was just some scam? Yes, I was.

I'm not sure how, or what, the CQC did but it certainly managed to contact this organisation and, as a result, the CQC rang me to say I would not be hearing any more about the matter, apparently it was the automated system they use for sending out invoices every month that had been at fault.

---

**Personal Reflection:** It takes a human being to programme these systems in the first place and, surely, when people no longer use a care home, in terms of moving to another, or on their demise, or for any other reason, the person responsible for this should make sure the name is deleted from the data automated system. As far as their lack of response to my telephone calls and letters over five years went, their behaviour highlights their arrogance and lack of feelings towards the family, let alone to the vulnerable people they care for.

---

**There's a Frog in the Basement: Strange Encounter** Embarking on the one hundred and sixty mile round trip to my parents' house, traffic was busy that day but still the sun was shining. Our visit was social but, more importantly, it was to check they were both okay. With Dad having Alzheimer's, which was now progressing, we were constantly worried about him and about my mother in terms of how she was coping, which was not very well.

When we arrived, my mother was a bit perturbed.

"What's wrong?" I asked.

She told me that Dad had been out that morning, and he was a long time. He went to the bank, because he said he had an appointment to see them to check his account, and he was going to get some cash back.

"But he does not know how to use the cash machine," I replied.

Mum said, "I don't even think he has been to the bank. I asked him when he got home, about half an hour ago, where he had been, and he said he couldn't remember."

"Well, did he have any cash on him?" I enquired.

"Yes, but I'm not sure how much."

"So he must have used the cash machine then."

What Mum told me next was deeply alarming. "Not long after he got in, I was in the kitchen." Which was where we all were now talking, a large driveway and garden occupied the front of the house surrounded by trees and a large garden at the back. It was a beautiful location that they'd retired to and only six minutes away from the beach.

"I was busy in the kitchen when I noticed a stranger walking around."

"What did you do?"

"I didn't really know what to do. I didn't go out, I just watched. He was looking at the house, and then he just disappeared."

I decided to ring the bank to see if Dad had had an appointment and if he'd attended. I was told, by the staff, that Dad did have an appointment but never turned up, so I asked them if Dad had been in the bank to get cash back from the cashier and was told no, so that left us thinking how on earth did Dad get his cash back?

I went into the lounge to talk to Dad, his face lit up with a welcoming smile, and I gave him a big hug and kiss.

"Hi Dad, are you okay?"

"I'm fine love, fine."

"Have you been out today?"

"No, I don't think so. Have you?"

"Yes, driven over from Leeds to see you and Mum. Have you

been to the bank, Dad?"

"No," he said.

"Not even to get some cash back?"

"Oh yes," he said. "I didn't know how to use that thing on the wall," he proceeded to take his wallet out of his pocket. "It's all in here though."

"What is?"

"A number, I write it on my wallet." I was shocked to see that Dad had written down all his bank details and PIN number actually on the leather of his wallet. "There was young man at the wall, and I asked him to help me."

"Oh no, Dad, you didn't."

Dad looked at me and said, "Why? What's up?"

"You don't give strangers your bank details. Did this person get your money out for you?"

"Yes," he said.

We could only assume that this person was the same one who Dad had spoken to and that my mum had seen walking into the garden, assuming that he had followed Dad home. I checked that their accounts were all okay and alerted the bank. This situation could have had a very different ending in terms of my dad's safety at the time, my mother's safety afterwards and financially.

**What Now?:** Jay claims Housing Benefit; I have also made sure that the contents of his home are insured. The council have a contract with an insurance company, so Jay's insurance is paid through that. The confusion arises when the rent account statement comes through from the council, but states the amount he is paying monthly for his insurance. I wonder why this is on a rent account statement, when a] he does not pay rent, and b] the monies are for insurance and not rent. When I first saw one of these rent account statements I queried it with the council and asked why couldn't it just be called insurance? I was told that it was just the way the system worked. This was not clear at the onset, which meant I had to query it by making a telephone call, so I could explain it to Jay.

---

**Care Homes**

**What it is Really Like Being a Relative for a Loved One in a Care Home**

**Lived Experience 9**

When the time came for my loved ones to move into a care home, I discovered it was not going to be as easy as I thought it would be, neither emotionally or physically.

First of all, it is not the easiest decision to make and yet, very often, it is the only decision one can take that is going to help. My parents made their own choices about where they lived and how they lived; they made their own decisions on moving, although they would discuss their plans of a move to a new location, and new home, with the family.

I always said, "If this is what you want and you are both going to be happy, go for it." Then through sudden and unexpected mental and/or physical ill health, the decision-making, like 'the ball in your court', is critically passed to the family about what happens next.

The whole procedure of looking for a care home, clearing out the existing family home, along with moving poorly parents, is a daunting prospect, especially when they are still detained in hospital. Decisions had to be made with each item of their personal belongings and furnishings in order to decide what they would no longer use or need. I felt like I was intruding into their personal space, the home they had loved for many years and the home in which many happy times were had.

The care home you choose is going to be your loved one's home for the rest of their lives; there are so many aspects we had to consider when choosing one, for example, it has to be appealing, comfortable, clean and pleasant, along with a good reputation and reports of excellence. My thoughts, as I looked around a care home, were; would I want to live here? Is it welcoming and effective, peaceful, does it have a hairdresser and chiropodist and will it meet my loved one's needs?

All this took serious thought and more, yet appraising was instrumental in being able to confirm and conclude that my loved ones were going to be safe, contented and happy, in addition to eating regular and well-balanced meals. A home in which they could still enjoy activities and trips out, all with the important presence and companionship of other residents.

Now, finally settled in a care home that had all of the above, including a lovely bedroom with an en suite, which Mum had insisted on having, she was happy. In some ways, I was sad, heavy-hearted, that my loved ones' lives would end in a care home and not in their own home where they really wanted to be.

In my positive frame of mind, I had peace of mind that they were being well looked after by professional staff and qualified nurses, and, without this sounding like I had been inconvenienced in any way whilst Mum was living with us, which I was not, we had a little more free time, and privacy from not having to have carers and professionals calling at the house all the time for physiotherapy, or resources like a commode etc. being delivered or long trips to the warfarin clinic, which just made Mum anxious.

Of course, I still did all the paperwork and accounts that were needed for my parents, but I was reassured that her medication and laundry was being taken care of in the home.

However, on our regular visits, Mum would say, "Will you look in the wardrobe?" Okay. I looked in the wardrobe.

"What am I looking in here for, Mum?"

"I can't find anything," she replied.

"What is it you are looking for?"

"Everything," she said. I quickly realised that what she really wanted me to do was to tidy her wardrobe.

I would take every item of clothing out of the wardrobe, of which she had far too many, and some she would never wear at all. I would show her each item, one by one, and ask her if she still needed it, did she still wear it, did she still want it? Then it would all go back in except the cardigans and other articles that had somehow strayed into the wardrobe that should have been in a drawer.

"I need a couple of new cardigans," she said. I knew exactly how many cardigans she had before I even opened the draw.

"There are at least eighteen cardigans in here," I replied.

"None of them fit me," she said. So, we went through all those, and then it would be underwear and footwear. I always got her what she asked for, and my heart went out to her, thinking how I would feel if I could not go for a leisurely trip to look at different items and shop for my own clothes. Mum always appreciated and liked the items I purchased for her and that made me happy.

Tidying the wardrobe, monitoring clothes, giving staff back the clothes that were not my mother's but somehow ended up in her wardrobe, and vice versa, buying new and checking her toiletries stock were all part of a day's work when we visited once a week or more. Communication is important with staff in the home, and together the manager would sit down with us and go through the care plan, checking that all was up to date, and for us to be kept up to date with what medication she was on. Mum was happy, therefore we were.

> **Personal Reflection**: We had visits where she would just complain about everything. Once an auxiliary nurse in a hospital, until she retired, where, in those days the matron ruled with a rod of iron and rotas where strictly followed, Mum's memories of those days were still with her and she would often say, "I haven't seen matron today, or matron's on holiday, but sister's in. Everything has changed here, hardly anybody is here now, and the ones that are have private flats." The content of her conversation bore no resemblance to the reality of the home at all.

There were sad and distressing visits too, especially when Mum started to suffer with acute delirium. It started when she said that she did not want to sleep in her bed any more, because each end of the bedhead had turned inwards towards her, so close it was around her neck, strangling her. On another occasion, she was lying in bed, where she could see the wardrobe which was against the opposite wall, she was so upset and frightened when she recalled that the previous night the wardrobe had started to move forwards and then backwards and forwards again, each time leaning more and more towards her, she said she thought it would crash down on top of her.

We had happy visits at the care home, where we could sit and chat and look at the 'good old days' photos I had on my phone, this would awaken her senses, stimulate her memory, thereby prompting her to tell us the story behind the pictures that span before and across the family's lives. She'll tell us about the therapy dogs that have been in and how she strokes and talks to them. She tells us that it is a delight to have seen and heard the school children singing Christmas carols for the residents. Despite Mum's delirium and confusion, we knew she was being well cared for.

If we know what to look for in a care home, we can make the correct decisions about which one is suitable for our loved ones. There is a great deal of information on the internet which gives guidance on how to choose a care home. It really is worth doing this kind of research if you and your family are contemplating this move in the future.

**There's a Frog in the Basement: Am I glad to see you, love.**
After receiving a call from the care home to say that my dad had fallen and had been taken into hospital again, not all the staff were sure whether or not Dad had hit his head so, to be on the safe side, they called the ambulance. I referred to my dad's wishes, that he did not want to be in hospital whatever the circumstances, he had stipulated many times that when the time came he wanted to stay in the home and be cared for in peace and quiet.

When we arrived at the hospital, Dad was standing at the entrance of the cubicle he had been allocated, when really he should have been lying down on the bed.

On seeing me he said, "Am I glad to see you, love. I want to go home."

I said, "I know you do, Dad, and we are going to take you home."

One of the nurses came up to us, and Dad said to her, "This is my daughter and her husband, and they have come to take me home."

I asked to speak to a senior nurse or the consultant after explaining that we needed to take Dad back to the care home, and there was nothing they could do for him at the hospital because Dad was already on the Gold Standard Framework.

As I was talking to the nurse, another nurse walked into the cubicle. My husband called to me and said, "She's come to take his bloods."

I said to the nurse, "He's not having them done, because I am taking him back to the care home."

At that moment the consultant arrived and, before I had chance to say anything, he said, "You know, if that were my dad, I would do exactly the same as you. Even if he has fallen and hit his head, if there was a bleed on the brain, there is nothing we can do because he is too poorly and would not survive an operation." He went on, "Give me five minutes."

When the consultant came back to us, he said that he had made the necessary phone calls and that we could take Dad back home. I thought to myself here is a professional who is talking sense, he did not put up any barriers that I feared I might have to challenge, and he could see the best course of action for Dad.

"Come on, Dad, we are going home."

"Thank you, love," he said as he held my hand to steady himself.

**What Now?:** It was Christmastime, and we had booked a

Christmas dinner at a local restaurant for all the family. Mum and Dad were in different care homes, at the time, and both were really looking forward to a get-together.

Dad was suffering from Alzheimer's; he really wasn't sure what was going on, although he was pleased to see his grandchildren. He wasn't saying very much, another indicator that Dad's condition was worsening. His little jokes and jollity on these occasions were definitely missing.

At times, Dad could get very angry and aggressive, which was immensely distressful to witness, when all his life he was such an amicable and sociable man, one whose skill, intelligence and astuteness led him to running his own business. We knew the little things that would upset him, the worst one being when the party was over and we had to take him back to the care home. We approached the moment as light-heartedly as possibly but with trepidation.

Laden with large and small Christmas presents and copious amounts of Christmas cards that had been exchanged between the families, we made our way to the car. My sister took my mum back to her care home, and we took Dad back to his.

He kept asking where we were going, and I said, "We are going back to the home, Dad." It wasn't a long journey but long enough for him to start getting worked up about it, although he wasn't getting angry, more upset. He said he did not want to go back to the care home; he wanted to go to his own home. We knew he did, we felt his angst, his sorrow and sadness, but we knew that the care home was the right place for him to get the care he needed.

When we arrived at the home, I walked in with Dad, who was getting more and more agitated. I carried all the presents whilst one of the male carers, who I have to say, was a man with a great deal of compassion and integrity and a genuine respect for his residents, helped me down to Dad's room.

I sat on the bed with Dad and took the presents out of the bag, reminding him who they were from. I asked him where he wanted me to put the presents, but he did not answer me. I passed the first one to him, he took if off me and held it, then I passed the second present to him and he took that off me, when suddenly he threw them across the room, he got the bags with the other gifts and started throwing them at me and shouting.

"Take them with you, I don't want any of them, I would rather die than be like this. I'm going to kill myself."

By this time, I was distraught and in tears, I just wanted my dad to be happy and to be with us all at Christmas. It had not turned out that way and maybe I'd made the wrong decision. The male nurse, who had been with us five minutes ago, must have heard the shouting and immediately came into see if everything was alright. He told me he would settle Dad down, so I left the care home terribly upset but knowing he was in good hands.

---

**Corporate Business**

**Mobile Phones**

**Lived Experience 10**

**Talks about the problems a carer can encounter when sorting problems out for their loved one**

*'Sorry we can't speak to you unless your son is with you.'* (Approx. 2015)

I went to the mobile phone company to sort out my son's account. Jay had been to town with a friend and had decided to take a contract out on a new phone, when he already had one. That was nine months ago, and I am still dealing with the aftermath of this situation. His new contract is costing £40 a month. How does he pay for two phones? He cannot. What can I do about it? I rang the company and explained the situation. They told me that because I was with the same company and my contract had expired, I could take over Jay's contract, that way he was not paying for two contracts.

If I chose not to do that, Jay would have an £88.00 cancellation fee to pay, so the first option sounded like a good idea. I agreed to take over the old contract. The company told me to ring back when my husband was with me, as he was the first named on the bank account, they would then take the bank details and change it all over.

When I rang back to do just this, the member of staff on the phone said, "Oh, we can't do that for you, we are not allowed to." Frustration was building rapidly, having again been given the wrong information from companies where staff were not knowledgeable in their company's procedures. So I rang again the day after, hoping to speak to someone who knew what he/she was doing and repeated the whole story yet again.

"That's okay," said the woman, "I will do it for you now," and proceeded to cancel the contract, as well as the direct debit, on Jay's old phone and swapped it to my name. She took all the bank details needed from the account, without my husband having to be there. Thank goodness for that, that's sorted. Oh no, it was not.

The following month, nothing had changed on Jay's account. I rang again and explained the situation.

I was told, "No, nothing has changed over or been cancelled," said the woman. "We can't do that." How could a person blatantly lie to me on the phone saying that she was changing the account and cancelling one, I heard her tapping away at the keys whilst she was doing it, more like she was doing something totally different like writing an email to a friend?

I wasn't just frustrated, I was absolutely fuming. How hard could it be to sort the problem out? I could not believe what I was hearing.

"The only thing you can do is to get a new SIM card for the old phone. On the other hand, you can cancel your son's contract which will cost you £80.00." [Inner thoughts] *We did not want a new SIM card for his old phone, he has just bought a new phone. What on earth is going on?*

"I am a carer, I am trying to sort this problem out for my son. I do not want a SIM card for his old phone, nor do I want a SIM card for my phone. I cannot be without a phone even for a few hours, let alone whilst the whole procedure takes place, like waiting for the card to come through the post."

I was so fed up of being lied to, dealing with staff who did not know what they were talking about, and staff making it appear that they were doing something to help when clearly they were not.

"Cancel it," I said, "just cancel it."

"Okay, if that is what you want us to do." [*That is not what I wanted them to do.*] "We will forward an invoice for the cancellation fee," but it never arrived. So I'm right back to square one after nine months, it beggars belief. The bank statement the following month showed that the company had taken £88.00 from it.

Did the story end there? No, I am afraid it did not. You can imagine my horror when I received email notification that my son's mobile phone bill was now ready, and the total cost was £150.00. I immediately went online to look at the bill in more detail.

Despite the company knowing that I was Jay's deputy through the Court of Protection, I could not access the bill online. I made numerous phone calls to the company about why I could not access this account, along with several live chats. One of the live chats went like this:

I typed out the full details of the problem and waited.

[Typing]

We cannot talk to you. Is your son there?

[Me typing]

No he is not.

[Typing]

Well, we can't help you. Is he available to take part in a three-way telephone conversation?

[Typing]

No, he is not.

[Typing]

Sorry, we cannot help.

[Typing]

Do you know anything about caring? Do you know what a deputy through the Court of Protection is? (COP) You cannot ignore a COP when I have authorisation through the courts to deal with his affairs, it is a legal document.

[Typing]

I can put you through to my manager.

[Typing]

Thank you. That would be useful.

[Typing]

This is the manager; please give me time to read your live chat from the beginning.

[Typing]

Okay. Thank you.

[Typing]

I can give you your son's password; it is the username that is being rejected?

[Typing]

Well I already have that, but go ahead, let me know what you have got. Can you do anything else?

[Typing]

That is all I can do.

Live chat ended. Have a good day.

I will not repeat what I said into the air at home to that comment.

I went back online. Did it work? No, it did not. My last port of call for help was to visit the mobile phone shop concerned, so off I went. Having arrived there, I once again explained the whole of the circumstances to one of the staff. He said he would have to get the manager. I showed them the legal document for COP (Court of Protection) to prove that I was a carer with this responsibility.

"Well," said the manger after repeating my soliloquy again. "In order to try and sort something out, we will need photo identification."

"What, you mean my photo ID?"

"No," said the manager, "your son's."

"But I have this legal document to prove I am who I say I am, and I have photo ID. Why do you need my son's photo? Is a photo ID more important and valid than the legal deputy through the Court of Protection document?"

There was no answer.

"Why do you need a photo of my son? Do you take photos of everyone when they come into the shop to buy a new phone and contract?"

"No, we do not take photos. We need it for identification," he replied.

"Have you got a photo of my son?" I asked.

"No."

"So what good will my son's photo ID be to you? How will a photo help in identification when you have not met my son and do not even know what he looks like?"

There was silence, a puzzled look on his face. (Ever seen this advert? – *Not made from wheat, made from oats instead – just call it Oatibix*.) Suddenly the penny dropped about what a stupid and senseless question he had just asked.

After a few seconds I said, "I have all the papers to confirm who I am, including the COP document. This is an issue I have been trying to sort out for months; it has cost money and a phenomenal amount of time, and time-wasting. What are you going to do about it?"

Finally, and without even looking at his papers, the manger sat down with me at the computer and, before long, he had me up and running online with a service username and a password. Now I could get access to the account, I would be able to check and monitor Jay's future bills. How hard was that?

---

**Personal Reflection**: What an ordeal. Why does this happen? This problem, like so many others, winds a carer up when we already have enough to cope with in life. Please listen to me properly, your full attention. Don't make promises you cannot keep. Stop making excuses just to get us off the phone line. Know how your business works, especially when you are dealing with the public and carers. Deal with the problem and resolve it for the customer. I was once waiting in line in the bank, when a guy in the queue

---

who was on his mobile, and not quiet, but definitely angry about an issue, was obviously talking to a mobile provider (I know this because after his long, and getting nowhere, call he yelled the mobile provider's name, followed by, "... you are totally useless and I will not be using you again."), I knew exactly how he felt.

Barriers put up. How many of them do carers jump over in a lifetime?

- What could have been done or said by staff to resolve this situation?
- How could the telephone conversations have been improved?
- Do you feel the staff had the correct knowledge and understanding of policy and procedures?
- How can we improve practice in corporate business in these situations?
- What information can you share with the professionals in order to get a clearer picture of what the carer is going through?
- Why do you think it took so much time to resolve this situation?
- Do you think the staff helped, if so, in what way?

**Quote:**

*Staff: There's no need to get angry and upset.*

*Me: I wouldn't be angry and upset if you did your job properly.*

**There's a Frog in the Basement: Emergency** After another busy day of caring, practically and emotionally, I was now at home, washing was in the machine, there was paperwork to do, and I had no energy to do it. Starting paperwork at this time in the evening meant not being able to unwind for an hour or so and then I would be late to bed. So I decided that this task could wait until tomorrow, and unwinding and going to bed got the vote.

At 9 p.m., I went to bed and started to read my book. It is a good way to fall asleep quickly; book still in my hand at an angle and glasses askew. There was peace and quiet, I was drifting off with thoughts of sunny skies, sandy beaches and the sound of lapping waves, when I was woken by someone singing '(I Can't Get No) Satisfaction' and it was not my husband. *My phone!* I thought waking with a start, which sits habitually every night on my bedside table. The display told me it was twelve minutes past midnight, and it was the care home ringing.

"Hello?" I said.

"Hi, is that Annie?"

"Yes, it is."

"Just to let you know that we have rung for an ambulance for your dad, as he is having chest pains. The paramedics are with him at the moment." She went on to inform me which hospital they would take him to.

"Thanks for letting me know. I'll meet him at the hospital."

In all aspects of my caring world, my husband is always there for me, to support and comfort, and to talk to at any hour of the day or night when I cannot sleep. At times like this, he is usually up and dressed before I am fully awake. In less than half an hour, we were driving to the hospital. We arrived there, as my dad was just being transferred from the ambulance to A & E.

Many hours of waiting around and answering questions followed.

Finally, when we saw Dad, he said, "Where am I? What am I doing here? Where's my wife?" Severe Alzheimer's brings no respite to the person suffering from it or for their carer. In the case of my dad, he asked the same questions only seconds apart from the last question.

When he asked about Mum, I just said she was okay in the care home. I'd stopped reminding him that she had had a stroke, because it was as if he was hearing this news for the first time, and it shocked and upset him. I answered his questions as best I could in a reassuring way and to comfort him. After waiting eight hours, my dad was finally admitted to a ward where they said they would keep him in for observation and do more blood tests. My husband and I finally left the hospital for home at 9 a.m. the following morning, reassured by staff that Dad was safe and doing well, despite the fact that he had had a heart attack. This was the eighth one.

**What Now?:** On a separate occasion, my dad was in hospital for a week after having an operation on his leg to remove a massive sarcoma tumour. It was December, with Christmas fast approaching, and Dad was discharged on the 22nd December. Late on the 24th December, he was rushed back into hospital with a pulse of twenty-three, with another heart attack, this time far more serious.

Dad had a 'do not attempt resuscitation' (DNAR) form in his medical notes. What the hospital staff asked me next came as a shock.

"We would like you to revoke the DNAR to enable us to fit a pacemaker." Those of you who have been in this situation will know, only too well, what it feels like to be faced with this dilemma.

Do I revoke the DNAR, or do I comply with my father's wishes and keep the DNAR in place? After a long discussion with the registrar, I told her I was not happy about consenting to this request, as it would be going against my father's wishes, and I knew my sister would feel the same way.

I was told that if a pacemaker was not fitted there was nothing more they could do for Dad, and there would be no point in him staying at the hospital. After being furnished with all the facts, I rang my sister. I told her what I had been told.

"If we do not agree to this, they said there is nothing more they can do, and if we take him home in the car, he could end up dying in my arms."

The nurse then said, "Oh, no, we would keep him at the hospital."

"You just said there would be no point in keeping him at the hospital."

My sister then had a long conversation with the registrar, and she made it clear that she did not want to subscribe to their request. The registrar told us that if we said no to the rescindment of the DNAR, they would overrule our decision, under their classification of the 'best interest' of the patient, however, the DNAR would be put back in place after the operation.

Finally, we had to comply with the hospital, and the member of staff tore the DNAR up in front of me and threw it in the bin. Consequently, a pacemaker was fitted on Christmas Day. My father was discharged on Boxing Day. Less than a week later, he was admitted again with a heart attack.

It was pointed out to me at the hospital that although DNAR means do not attempt to resuscitate, it does not mean, do not attempt to care. At that time, he did not need resuscitation. I understand that a pacemaker keeps the beat of the heart going, however, it does not prevent heart attacks or a failing heart. It is still a controversial and ethical issue that is debated, to this day, in terms of: if the patient has a DNAR, it can be overruled by medical staff in the 'best interest' of the patient, despite the fact that the patient has a DNAR in place and regardless of the next of kin, with an LPA that covers health issues, trying to ensure that a loved one's wishes are adhered to. I also discovered that a patient without a DNAR can have one implemented by the hospital, in the 'best interest' of the patient, if nothing more can be done.

I have no doubt there are many debates, in cases like this, in terms of opposing or consenting, I however found this very confusing, as I thought that a DNAR meant that if my father had a heart attack and a dangerously low pulse that he would be made comfortable and allowed to have a natural demise.

Life is much more complex than we think until we are faced with the real situation. My dad, my husband and I were treated with courtesy and respect from the staff, as well as being given quality time to talk and ask questions put to senior staff, however, this was punctuated, at times, by quite surly and superior attitudes from other staff.

---

**Corporate Business**

**Better Banking for Carers**

**Lived Experience 11**

**Statement of Support by Dr Elaine McNichol – University Of Leeds**

Annie is a long-standing, valued member of our Patient and Public Involvement Group in the School of Healthcare at the University of Leeds. She has extensive experience as carer and, due to her excellent teaching and communication skills, she is able to share that experience in a way that brings issues to life and enables our nursing and social work students to gain valuable learning. Annie is a passionate advocate for service users and carers and well respected in the caring community for highlighting and trying to address the injustices that carers experience in trying to look after and manage the affairs of their loved ones, sometimes despite the system rather than supporting it.

The challenges of working with the banking system is similar to many of the large corporations that, despite providing the paperwork to demonstrate the legal right to manage a person's affairs, carers report that they are frequently 'blocked' from doing so. As a result, a simple task becomes a complex and frustrating one on top of the daily challenges that a unpaid carer faces.

*Please note: all information is correct at the time this took place, policies, procedures, laws and regulations may have changed since then.*

**Mind-Boggling Banking** – *You are blocked from using online banking for your son because you are using it illegally.*

I do not have to state the obvious to the millions of carers in this country that our caring role can be extremely rewarding and, at the same, formidable, yet we still continue to care for our loved ones because we are concerned about their well-being in pretty much all aspects of their lives. Carers and service users must be recognised and accepted, not alienated and disregarded, by any services. In this case, I was on the receiving end of illogical bureaucracy, along with belittling dialogue, that made me feel inadequate and made my mind boggle with contradictory directives.

Our caring passion drives us to make sure that those less fortunate than ourselves are not excluded or exploited by anyone, however, in this situation, it took me several years, with the help of professionals, to tell the banks that:

*"Why have you blocked me from managing my son's accounts*

*online?"*

*"Because you are using it illegally, and we don't have the systems to deal with a deputy through the Court of Protection."*

*"Why haven't you got the systems to deal with a person who holds a deputy role through the Court of Protection? I have been managing Jay's online accounts for the last year."*

*"You could be fraudulent."*

*"Why would I want to be fraudulent to my lovely son, who means the world to me, and needs help and support?"*

*"You cannot have two usernames, it is illegal."*

*"Well, if that is the case, you had better tell the staff at the branch, because they set it up for me."*

I had been using online banking for a year for my son, as a deputy through the Court of Protection. On the 16th February 2010, I logged in as usual and was declined access. The notice I saw on this page was that sometimes they have to close it down, and to try again, which I did, but to no avail. It suggested ringing the helpline number, which I did, and I explained that I had been denied access and asked them why. They said it was because I was using online banking illegally and that the username I had given would not pass security. They told me to call in at my local branch, with some identification, and they would sort it out for me. So I did.

The customer care advisor at the branch rang the helpline

for online banking and confirmed that I was who I said I was, and that I had shown her my driving licence and passport. Then I spoke to John, the person on the helpline. Again, I was told that they could not give me access using that username, because it was not valid and did not belong to me. I had to use the username that my son had. Jay did not have a username, because he does not use a computer and therefore is not linked up to the internet, does not go online, nor would he be able to fully understand the online banking procedure and the monitoring of his accounts.

John told me that they had a username for Jay. This was the first time I had heard that the bank had a username for Jay, so I asked him what it was; he said he could not tell me.

I said, "Well how can I access his accounts then, if you are saying on the one hand that I have to use Jay's service username, how can I use it when you won't tell me what it is?" I continued. "What is the solution to this problem then?"

John said, "I don't know." He just kept repeating that no one could have two service usernames for online banking and would not reinstate my online banking. I soon realised that jumping over this whopping embankment was going to be an uphill battle, to say the least.

This made dealing with my son's finances very difficult. Normally, after receiving his benefits into the main current account, I would then transfer his daily money into his personal account. Therefore, because I was not allowed access to his account any more, I had to go to the cash machine to take out his weekly money and take it up to him, giving him the cash he needed for the day. This was a ridiculous and time-consuming situation, in addition to an already busy, and established, caring schedule.

I went to my local bank again and told them what had happened. They could not understand why online services were saying this, as I had been using online banking for a long time, and my local branch had a copy of the Court of Protection (COP). They suggested I phoned online banking again, from the branch, and I spoke to Phillip.

Once again, I explained that I had been using online banking for a year now. I asked him how he had got a service username from Jay, and he replied that he hadn't. Jay's was the same service username that I had, the one I had been using all along, and the one that was declined.

He went on to say that he could see on the records that staff at the branch had helped me set up online banking, that they should never have done this, and had no right to do this. We were just having a loop dialogue throughout which was very confusing. I asked Phillip if he had any understanding of what a deputy through the Court of Protection's role is, and how important this service was to me in order to keep Jay's accounts managed correctly.

He said, "I know what I am doing at this end."

He told me I should not be using online banking for my son, as I was doing this illegally by having two service usernames and, in addition to that, that my son could access this account at any time. I pointed out that firstly, Jay would not access the account, as he did not have a computer and would not even know where to start with the online procedure required and secondly, hypothetically, if I had my own business, I would have a business service username and password for that account. I would also have my own personal account which would have a separate service username and password and thirdly, I managed my son's account, thereby having yet another service username and password, in which, as I had been doing, I managed his account legitimately as a deputy through the Court of Protection.

Whichever way I looked at this unexplained problem that they had stumbled upon, I still could not understand why they could not understand what I was talking about. They did not offer any solution, in order to rectify the matter, but just kept repeating that I was using that account fraudulently.

I asked them if they knew of the Office of the Public Guardian, the governing office that legally approved the Court of Protection rights, what a deputy of the Court Protection was, along with the roles and responsibilities of such a post. I also asked them if they knew what an unpaid carer was and their roles in society.

The only response to these questions was, "The Office of the Public Guardian tells us what to do."

I rang the Office of the Public Guardian and asked them what information they give to banks in terms of LPAs, OPGs etc., and they told me that they advise banks of all these legal contracts and changes that arise, but they did not tell them how to bank. All my other questions, I am afraid to say, fell on deaf ears.

I explained to the bank that taking out a COP is not done on a whim, it needs careful consideration and it is costly. When the document is completed, it is then passed to the courts for acceptance. Once this is done, it is given a legal and law-abiding stamp of approval, which means that the courts have legally deemed the applicant to be the responsible and appropriate adult to act for their loved one as a deputy through the Court of Protection.

I told them I was making this call from the local branch and that the manager was at my side, and he himself, could not believe what he was hearing. He even spoke to Phillip and told him that, from their end, my username had not been blocked or stopped in any way and was fine to use, adding that my husband and I had been customers of the bank for years and he could vouch for our good name and trustworthiness.

After nearly forty minutes of getting nowhere, I asked to speak to his manager, as this young man's manner and attitude was unhelpful and, in my opinion, extremely unprofessional. He told me to hold, so I held. I held for about seven minutes and then he cut me off. The manger of the branch supported me with this issue and did so with utmost professionalism and courtesy.

Distraught and upset, I went home, stunned and angered that I had been accused of fraudulence. I was made to feel like a charlatan. Was that what they really thought of me? I had abided by the law all my life, and now I was being looked upon as some sort criminal, not even worthy enough to be listened to. A cheat I am not, and that is because I have been brought up by two good parents who taught me right from wrong and good from bad.

My dad used to say, "Don't let anyone take advantage, exploit or manipulate you in any way, stand up for your rights, Annie." My moral values and social skills came from my parents, and I have lived my life by their traditional wisdom, moral and social values, making me the person I am today.

The one thing I have discovered, within my many years of lived experiences in caring, is injustice, it always seems to be there, lurking around every corner, ready to jump out at you when least expected.

When we care for our loved ones, we have to ensure that their voices are heard and, as carers, make sure their needs are met in every aspect of life. Why? Because we want justice. I was irritated, disappointed and thoroughly hacked off from being treated like an incompetent castaway. So now there was only one thing to do and that was to devote however many months it took to fight the banks on this preposterous, discriminatory violation of my right to be my son's deputy through the Court of Protection and my son's right to have a personal bank account.

I had already made a verbal complaint and embarked on writing my first official complaint to the bank. In addition to this, I had already started to keep a record of telephone conversations, dates, days, times, names, along with what had been said in answer to my questions. I kept all correspondence and documents in order to build up a file on the case for Better Banking for Carers.

By keeping a case file, I was also ready to give it to my solicitor and MP when the need arose and, needless to say, it did. One of the aspects in applying for a lasting power of attorney in finances and/or in health, Court of Protection, or similar is that it has to be applied for whilst the person it is for still has capacity to choose the person they would like to appoint. However, I was told, from a bank, that once these documents have been registered with the Office of the Public Guardian then online access cannot be granted for donor or attorney.

When we are expected to use modern-day technology for many aspects in life, it is important to recognise the needs of carers who want to use online banking regardless of what legal document they hold in terms of a deputy through a Court of Protection order, lasting power of attorney or similar, none of these legal documents should be made exempt from online banking, as it was in my case.

A lasting power of attorney (LPA) is a document that lets you (the 'donor') appoint one or more people (known as 'attorneys') to help make decisions or to make decisions on your behalf. [*Gov. uk*] The LPA may give you permission to make decisions, while the donor still has mental capacity to make their own decisions, if it does not, then you can only start making decisions when they do not have capacity. From experience of dealing with three people's health and finances, I found it extremely helpful and useful to have the LPA in property and financial affairs as well as health and welfare. Under these circumstances, I pointed out the importance of carers having the need to be a deputy and having access to online banking, if they so wish.

A person who does not have full capacity has a far greater need for a loved one/main carer to be an attorney, whereas the person who has full capacity, like my mother and father had, asked me to be a lasting power of attorney for them. It is pretty obvious that some individuals are able to express what they would like, whilst others cannot.

At the time my complaint was made, the facts and figures available from the Mental Health Trust, Mind and Carers UK stated that over two million people lacked mental capacity which impaired them from making decisions, whether this was due to dementia, learning difficulties, brain injuries or other mental health conditions, **the law allows other people to act on their behalf.**

The Office of the Public Guardian began in 2007 and, according to statistics, at the time of writing, they handled over 90,000 applications. At the end of 2018, over 3.4 million LPAs, and 150,000 enduring power of attorneys were on their register, in addition to supervising 59,000 court-appointed deputies and, for the first time, they were now supervising court-appointed guardians of missing people as detailed with the Guardianship (Missing Persons) Act of 2017.

To qualify for power of attorney to access online banking, the attorney must have full power of attorney i.e. the authority to access all the donor's accounts including any that may be opened in the future.

Jay has several accounts and, as a deputy through the Court of Protection, I am authorised to manage them. However, I was told that the online facility could not be applied to joint accounts. The customer service I received was abysmal, in terms of little and poor knowledge of the business they were running, certainly no happy face emojis for attitude and social skills, and an obvious lack of understanding of the carer's role.

By not allowing carers, who have painstakingly read and filled in applications, to apply to act on their loved one's behalf and basically follow the correct procedure to become an attorney or similar, for the sole reason of providing a stable and consistent daily living routine where money is concerned, they are not only ostracising the two million carers or more but discriminating against them as well. Carers rely on the professionals to help us ensure that the cared for person's wishes for the future are carried out.

I spent hours researching every possible line of enquiry in this case, to establish facts for disability rights from the Equality Act, internal policies, systems and procedures on online banking, facts from every issue prominent to this complaint. This included the general industry practice which stated that any person suffering with a physical or mental health disability should be able to access any service that the able-bodied could. This statement, amongst all my research, was the most crucial and a driving factor in order to make my case, along with the fact that carers and service users in this instance were being discriminated again.

**February 2010**

I wrote my first letter of complaint outlining the issues that I referred to earlier in this Lived Experience, in addition to asking why online banking did not recognise carers who were deputies through the Court of Protection. And why did the banks not recognise carers in their own right? Following the complaints procedure, I liaised with the manager of my local branch, therefore, the first letter went to him. I was sent a reply, which was not at all satisfactory, and therefore I sent a reply stating why I was dissatisfied with their first response.

**March 2010**

I received a letter from the bank thanking me for my visit to the branch. It stated that they understood I was unhappy with the following:

Bank: You have Court of Protection for your son, and you are unhappy with it.

Me: Yes, I have, but I am not unhappy with it unless someone takes it away from me.

Bank: You use online service for your son's accounts to ensure that his finances are kept in good order.

Me: Yes, I do, and I am not unhappy about doing this for him. I am unhappy, because I have not been allowed the resources to do it with.

Bank: I have been told by the online help desk that you should not have access to your son's online account.

Me: Yes, I was.

Bank: You feel that this is discrimination against people who have Court of Protection.

Me: Yes, I do.

Bank: When you rang the online help desk, you found them to

be condescending and unhelpful.

Me: Yes, I did.

Why are they repeating all the statements I have made to them, back to me, in a reply letter without any substance? The letter went on to say that they would like to apologise for the poor service I had received from the online help desk, and my comments had been passed to the relevant department for their consideration.

I was told, at the start of the complaint, that the online banking service was a separate entity from the bank's branches, it continued that whilst they fully accepted that I had legal authority to maintain my son's accounts they, regrettably, did not offer online banking access to those customers who held Court of Protection for a customer. I had been using online banking for my son, as deputy through the Court of Protection, for a year when all this came to light.

They fully understood how stressful and difficult such a situation was, and they were empathetic to the situation I found myself in. They were therefore concerned to learn of the conflicting advice I had received from staff, going on to say that if a customer held a power of attorney (POA) then online access could be granted, and online access would be given to both the attorney and the donor.

I reiterated that I had Court of Protection, why was online banking given to just people who held power of attorney? What did it matter whether it was for lasting power of attorney, or Court of Protection, that person was still the person who was responsible for looking after another person's affairs and, more often than not, the carer? Online access, it was stated, would be given to the donor as well. The donor is the person who needs the help. It appears that the donor must not have any mental health impairment but must have full capacity of their mental health.

There are many people who have this role and many of the people being looked after have mental health problems. The donor may well have the capacity to understand what the attorney is taking out and agree to it, but it does not mean to say that the donor has the capacity to fully manage their finances or understand online banking.

My father had Alzheimer's, he was initially just forgetting things in a small way, however, he was able to understand what LPOA meant and that is what he wanted, so he signed the forms with my mother. I was the attorney for both of them. When we got home, he could not remember that we had been to the solicitors.

However, if a power of attorney (POA) has been granted with the Court of Protection (COP) order, this is usually because a court has deemed the account holder incapable of managing their finances, and it does not mean that he can't tell me he is hungry. *Before applying for COP, I spoke to my solicitor to find out what it entailed and whether he would apply for this for me. He told me I could apply online and that it would save money, so that is what I did.*

In March 2010, I sent my second letter of complaint in response to the bank's previous letter. This again went through the manager of the local branch. So, having exhausted the first part of compliance to the complaint procedure, it was then passed to a senior member of staff at head office. I had more letters, and I wrote yet more replies, in addition to making numerous visits to my local branch.

It was obvious that this situation was going round in circles, especially when I went to the branch to sort out one of Jay's accounts, not a major task one would think, however, after being in the office for an hour, the member of staff said to me, "I can't sort that account for you because you are a deputy through Court of Protection."

"Yes," I replied, "and you have all the legal documents to verify that. I have come to the branch to do this, because I am not allowed to use online banking. It seems to me that, right at this moment, my deputyship does not even allow me to come into the branch to sort out an account."

"Sorry," she said.

"Right back to square one then," I said, and that was my polite reply. "Right," I said, "I have had about as much as I can take with this problem, and I am now going to make this public," and I walked out of the bank.

Following this visit, I went home and wrote to the ombudsman in addition to setting up a meeting with my MP.

**6th August 2010 – Financial ombudsman's first reply**

*The bank has acted unfairly and unreasonably in removing*

*Annie's internet banking access to administer her son's account. In order to settle this complaint, the bank should now provide Annie with internet banking facilities to administer her son's accounts. Prior to the bank becoming aware that she is a deputy through the Court of Protection on behalf of her son's finances, the bank withdrew Annie's access to internet banking for her son's account. This has effectively prohibited Annie from managing her son's finances in accordance with the COP.*

*The bank's policy, from April 2009, states that its systems are unable to provide internet banking access for a deputy such as Annie. The bank stated that there have been systems put in place to get around this problem in the past. Other banks provide internet access facilities for deputies and this bank's stance is not consistent with general industry practice.* [It went on to suggest that the bank might have broken the law requiring equal treatment for able and disabled customers.] *We have been unable to resolve your complaint informally to the satisfaction of both sides because the bank did not agree with the decision reached by the adjudicator.*

When I asked the ombudsman what would happen now, I was told that failure of an organisation to comply with the adjudicator's/ombudsman's decision was enforceable in court. The ombudsman would now need to review the whole case again and formally make a final decision. This involved looking at the entire case file again and taking into account all the comments and information that had been provided during the investigation.

## November 2010 – The ombudsman's final decision

## Complaint

*Mrs Dransfield complains that, as appointed deputy for her son under a Court of Protection order, the Halifax stopped her having access to online banking. She further complains about the way the bank has dealt with the matter.*

## Our initial conclusions

*The adjudicator recommended the complaint be upheld. He did consider that the Halifax had treated Annie unfairly by removing online banking access. Not only had it accepted there had been ways to get around the situation in the past, but the bank's approach was not consistent with general industry practice. The Halifax said this was just a matter of its own internal policy; its present systems did not allow online access where a Court of Protection order had been registered because it could not be restricted just to the deputy – the account holder could have access too. But it noted that Annie may incur inconvenience in moving the accounts and it offered her £100.*

## My final decision

*I have considered all that Annie and the Halifax have said and provided, in order to decide what is fair and reasonable in this complaint.*

*Annie had online access for about a year after the order was granted. She has outlined the frequent contact she had with her local branch about her son's accounts, how under the order she is personally responsible for his finances, how online banking is central to her managing the accounts and how her son is not capable of using the internet.*

*There is nothing to stop the Halifax from giving Annie what she used to have, other than its policy and systems - where it seems the likelihood of her son misusing the facility is negligible. Also, the bank has obligations under the Equality Act to make 'reasonable adjustments' - I consider these to be just such circumstances. Moreover, our enquiries have shown that within Lloyds Banking Group, of which Halifax is a member - the facility Annie used to have, and seeks reinstating, can be made available.*

*I therefore find the fair outcome is for the Halifax to reinstate Annie's full online banking. I also consider she has been caused unnecessary distress and inconvenience for which she should be compensated. I find the bank's offer to be too low; I consider £300 to be fairer. My final decision is that I uphold this complaint.*

*Under the rules of the Financial Ombudsman Service, I am required to ask Annie either to accept or reject my decision in writing before the 9th December 2010.*

**February 2011**

My MP, Stuart Andrew, and the staff I liaised with at the Financial Ombudsman Service were so professional, efficient, helpful and understanding, explaining their procedure and what could be done, and all parties concerned were in frequent contact.

I had decided to make this issue public before this decision was made by the ombudsman. It was suggested, by a certain person (who I cannot name due to him moving and not being able to contact him for permission), that I ring a certain journalist on a particular paper who would be interested in my plight. When I rang the paper, the journalist I asked for was not in the office that day, however, the journalist who took my call took the story up. The following article continues the story.

**12th February 2011 – Case made public**

**Headlines by Richard Dyson,** Daily Mail, **12th February 2011:** "Mother blocked from disabled son's account despite damning report by Ombudsman"

*When Annie found she had been denied online banking access to her disabled son's Halifax bank accounts, she thought it was a technical problem that the bank would sort out swiftly.*

*Unfortunately, it turned into a year-long battle with Lloyds Banking Group, which owns Halifax, and prompted Annie to launch a campaign to improve the service that banks give the growing army of carers.*

*Annie, 56, from Leeds, cares full-time for 32-year-old Jay who has cerebral palsy. He has two accounts in his name, both of which Annie has authority to access granted by the Court of Protection in February 2009.*

*Annie says, "It is important for Jay to have financial independence. I oversee the accounts, but the money is his." It suited Annie, a former drama teacher, to operate the accounts online. That way she could make payments while ensuring Jay had access to money if, for instance, he was with his care support worker and needed money in an emergency.*

*For a year this worked smoothly, but last February the Halifax blocked Annie's access to Jay's accounts. When she phoned the help support number, she was told to go to her branch. The staff at the local branch knew her and were sympathetic, but they too hit a brick wall. Executives higher up the bank said that what Annie wanted was impossible.*

*Annie decided to fight and says, "Like all carers, I hadn't time to waste battling with bank bureaucracy. I wanted to show senior people within the bank that their decisions and systems made life harder for carers.*

*"Being involved with mental health organisations, I had great insight into the problems carers face when dealing with someone else's finances. It's a nightmare. I wanted to put it right." Lloyds rejected her complaints, forcing the matter into the hands of the Financial Ombudsman's Service.*

*The FOS sided with Annie. Last November, in a damning adjudication, it ordered Lloyds to restore her online access to Jay's accounts and pay £300.00 for unnecessary distress.*

*It said that nothing prevented the bank from offering online access other than its policy and systems. It went even further, suggesting the bank may have broken the law requiring equal treatment of able and disabled customers.*

*Amazingly, Lloyds ignored the FOS's verdict for three months. Only after* Financial Mail*'s involvement late last month did it* *restore Annie's access to Jay's accounts and apologise. Lloyds refuses to explain why Annie was denied access, why it forced her to use the FOS and why it ignored the ruling.*

*Worse, it refuses to say how it will treat other customers in Annie's position. Helen Weir, Lloyds boss of current accounts, has spoken about the need for bank staff to have authority to resolve complaints early. Yet when, 1.8 million a year, Weir was asked to comment on Annie's case, the request was declined.*

*The bank apologised for any inconvenience caused to Annie and said Annie's complaint had been highlighted at a very senior level.*

We were still in the House of Commons when, immediately after this debate, HBOS sent a message to my MP saying:

*We are very sorry for any inconvenience this caused to Annie and her son. We clearly failed to get this right first time. Annie has a valued and long-standing relationship with the bank, particularly with her local branch. We worked with Annie and found a solution, which works for her.*

*We recognise that customers have individual needs. We encourage colleagues to work with customers with disabilities, making adjustments that will enable them to fully access banking services wherever possible. We have a range of adjustments that we put in place for different groups of people. We understand the importance of getting things right for our customers and already have a specialist teams in place across Lloyds TSB, Halifax and Bank of Scotland to manage all Power of Attorney and Court of Protection requests.*

*We are investing in further training for colleagues over the coming months as part of our ongoing commitment to excellent customer service. If there is anything else I can do to help, please do not hesitate to get in touch.*

After my online banking had been reinstated, I had a follow-up call from the bank. They rang to find out if everything was okay. I asked them if they would do the same for other carers who I knew were experiencing the same problems. They said that this was a 'one-off' and they would not do it for anyone else.

"If you can do this for me, you can do it for all the other millions of carers who have, or are having, the same or similar problems as me using online banking." I was met with silence.

If the bank had not adhered to the ombudsman's decision the second time around, it would have been enforceable in court.

Richard Dyson's article continued:

*Three in five people will become a carer, most commonly of a partner, spouse or parent. Where there is cognitive impairment, carers frequently need to oversee their financial affairs and the most common way to manage this is to set up a lasting power of attorney. These must be set up while people still have mental capacity and can appoint attorneys themselves, and they take at least three months to register and are usually designed to become effective only later.*

*LPAs replaced Enduring Powers of Attorney in October 2007, however, a pre-2007 EPA remains valid.*

*It is different when the person you care for is already unable to manage, in these circumstances, the carer can be appointed as a deputy through the Court of Protection. Banks should recognise LPAs and deputies and help in the operating of accounts.*

Andrew Chidgey of the Alzheimer's Society *says, "Very often carers are met with bank cashiers who don't understand, or accept, the LPA. We'd like to see improvements across all banks in terms of staff training and more flexible systems."*

Financial Mail*'s campaign to improve services at Santander bank has unearthed dozens of cases where accounts operated under LPAs are mismanaged. "Most banks do correct errors," says Jean French, of charity Carers UK. "Yes, frustrations occur and banks could do better, but in most people's experience banks do take complaints regarding LPAs seriously," she says. [Richard Dyson for the* Daily Mail *and* Mail Online. *Last updated 12th February 2011]*

*Public Responses to the article: The following excerpts are published with permission from the authors. These responses refer to either the same online bank as mine or other banks.*

Déjà Vu: *Your story gave me a feeling of déjà vu. I eventually stopped writing to the ... after my mother suffered a stroke and I felt that to continue might prove pointless. Following your story, I have started again to request online access to my mother's accounts. What really makes my blood boil is the attitude of; we do not really give a damn about your problems, just let us have an easy life and let us continue to 'rip you off'.*

Long-Distance Caring: *My young brother aged fifty-one*

*years old, with a mental age of two, has very severe learning difficulties. I eventually and happily became a deputy through the Court of Protection for him. I have banked with the ... for many years and have several accounts with them. I deal with all of the accounts online. As a carer, this saves time of having to queue in branches or hang on the phone for ages with telephone banking. I thought it would be an easy process to open an account on behalf of my brother. Everything seemed to be alright at first. The bank had full knowledge of the Court of Protection. I was sent a letter to say that the type of account I wanted to open could not be given online access. I believe I was misled at the outset, as I was originally informed that online access would be available. I have had numerous discussions with the security department and it all comes down to a 'systems' issue, apparently. My brother never has any input into the account I manage for him, because he has never had the mental ability to do so and never will. The bank decrees this to be a potential security issue, suggesting that somehow or other he could gain access to all the online security codes and operate the account without my knowledge. He cannot even turn a TV on. He lives more than sixty miles away from me and is cared for 24/7 in accommodation by the Housing Association.*

*At least you got further than I did with operating online. The branch said "No problem" when I opened the account, it was about a week later I received a letter from its head office saying that due to a systems issue it would not be possible to operate the account online. What makes me so annoyed is that every time I have to do something manual on the account, involving either the branch or Head Office, I get a letter suggesting that I might like to operate the account online. Ironic and frustrating isn't it? When the banks are suggesting we go online and then will not* let us. *I do hope that when the bank has sorted out these systems we will not have these problems any more, we wait and see. If I can be of any assistance in your efforts, please do not hesitate to get in touch.*

Bureaucracy: *I opened an ISA account for my father using EPA. It took over an hour of bureaucracy at the local branch before we achieved what we wanted, however I am now being denied online access. I have concluded that banks are completely ignorant of these issues and high-handed. Best of luck with Better Banking for Carers and hope this is of some help.*

Our Loved Ones Deserve the Same Service as Everyone Else: *I read your article with interest, having come across very similar problems as you do. I seem to be hitting my head against a very solid brick wall. Not giving my son the same rights as everybody else seems unfair and discriminate. I would certainly add my name to your list when Better Banking comes to fruition for our children's rights.*

Online Banking IT – A Complete Shambles: *Just an update Annie from my perspective. Now ... have taken over the IT systems of ... they are supposedly allowing deputies to have internet access. However, the IT situation is a complete shambles. I have made two official complaints and received a small compensation. I am about to make my third official complaint, as it is still not sorted.*

*Hi Annie, Since my last email I have moved everything away from the ... to ... which I have found to be more helpful and understanding. I do not think that anything will happen to the customers' advantage, as I think the politicians are in the banks' pockets. Cynical I know but from my own experience... Thanks again for keeping me informed.*

Online banking and technology overall surrounds us in our everyday life, I remember Prime Minister David Cameron telling us that he wanted to see everyone with a PC and be online. My thinking, on this statement, is this and what most of us are aware of anyway is that not everyone can afford a computer, not everyone wants to use a computer, not everyone has the capacity to use a computer and, for the homeless in society, just having to use organisations that provide access to computers is difficult for them. He continued to say that *"cheques are being phased out"*, and banks tell us that *"banking couldn't be easier"*. I can very clearly state that this has not been my experience, and there is a long way to go before banking meets the varying needs of carers and their loved ones.

Through these experiences, it appears that persons wishing to do so can apply for a deputy through the Court of Protection, like I did, but were not told that banks do not offer online banking for this type of deputy.

Office of the Public Guardian: My experiences so far in dealing with the Office of the Public Guardian staff are that they are very approachable and helpful. When I spoke to them in connection with my online banking dilemma, they stated that they would go into corporate businesses to train staff on aspects of LPAs and deputies through a Court of Protection order if the company wished to do so.

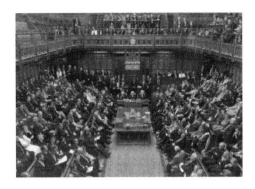

**2nd February 2012: Column 1111** – Debate in the House of Commons Carers and Online Banking.

Stuart Andrew {Pudsey} {Con}: These days we seem to talk a lot about banks and banking, and for many in the House it is nice that there is a profession slightly less popular than ours. Since notice was given on this debate, I have had Right Hon. and Hon. Members ask me what it was about and when I explained it, many of them gave examples of similar problems raised with them by their constituents. I am glad, therefore, to have been able to secure this debate.

All Members on both sides of the House value, and know the value of, carers in this country. There are almost 6 million carers in the United Kingdom – a staggering one in ten people – and, according to Carers UK, over the next 30 years their number will increase by 3.4 million. That is about a 60% increase. Some 1.25 million carers care for more than 50 hours a week. Indeed, carers are estimated to save the Government between £67 billion and £87 billion a year, and a 2011 report by the University of Leeds for Carers UK estimated that the economic value of the contribution made by carers in the UK is £119 billion per year. Bearing in mind our current deficit, those are staggering figures.

Before being elected, I worked in the hospice movement, and time and again I would see carers' hard work and dedication. I remember one father saying that if he got up for his child eight times in a night, he would think that he had had a good night's sleep. As MPs, we know the value of carers and the challenges they face, whether from those who visit us in our surgeries or from the visits that we make to organisations representing them.

Being a carer is about long hours and hard work, and because they are often caring for loved ones it is sometimes deeply emotional. They are an army of people whose dedication and compassion we should cherish. It is in that vein and spirit that I asked for this debate. In a decent country such as the UK, we should do all that we can to help improve the lives of carers and make things as easy as possible for them. I am delighted, therefore, that the Government have committed an extra £400 million to supporting respite support for carers, and I look forward to that money reaching the people who need it.

A few months ago, two constituents of mine, Mr and Mrs Dransfield, came to one of my surgeries. It was their story, and the fact that their experience is not isolated, that persuaded me to raise this issue today. Annie is the full-time carer of her 32-year-old son, who suffers from cerebral palsy and mental health issues. Like carers up and down the country, she helps and supports her son to manage day-to-day activities that I, for one, am fortunate enough to be able to do unassisted. For her son it is different. Annie has to help around the house, sort papers out and deal with other household issues. She also has to take management of his finances. In February 2009, she applied to be her son's deputy through the Court of Protection.

This was duly approved and, as a consequence, she was given access to her son's bank account at the local Halifax branch. The arrangement helps her son to be financially...

**2nd Feb 2012: Column 1112**

...independent, as the money that he is given is paid into his account and she merely ensures that it is managed correctly.

As we all lead increasingly busy lives, so our daily activities have had to change. As a consequence, many of the services offered by various institutions have maximised the use of new technology to help us. Online banking is a good example of that; indeed, it is something that I have come to rely on. So it was that Annie decided to use online banking for her son's account. She has explained why it is so important:

"As a carer, the ability to access my son's accounts online is invaluable. It means I don't have to make the journey to his bank and give him is money each day and it also gives me peace of mind. If he loses his money, or does not realise how much he has spent and has nothing to get home with or buy food with, he can call me and, in less than two minutes, I can transfer some extra cash in his account so that can get home safely or get something to eat."

To give him some independence and responsibility, Mrs Dransfield's son has a cash card account that she keeps topped up from his current account. That helps him with his daily routine, giving him the motivation to get up, go out and walk to get some cash.

That arrangement worked extremely well, until one day, Mrs. Dransfield tried to access her son's account and found that she was blocked from doing so. The cash machine also retained his card when they tried to use it. Naturally, she contacted the bank, only to be told that it was illegal to have two online usernames, despite Annie having the authority to manage her son's account. This started a long and time-consuming battle with her bank to have her access reinstated. The bank refused to back down. As a result, the case was referred to the Financial Ombudsman Service, which concluded that Annie was correct. In November, the FOS ordered the bank in its adjudication to reinstate her online access. The ombudsman found that the bank has obligations under the Equality Act 2010 to make 'reasonable adjustments' and that the fair outcome would be for the bank to restore her online banking in full. In addition, the ombudsman said that the bank should pay £300 for 'unnecessary distress' and that the only thing preventing access was the bank's policy and systems. I am sure that we would all agree that that was a sensible verdict.

Staggeringly, the bank ignored the Financial Ombudsman Service's verdict. Feeling desperate, Annie found that her only option was to turn to the media. Thankfully, the *Mail on Sunday* took up the story. It was only then that the bank took action and permitted her access to the account again. However, what is shocking is that, as I understand it, that resolution is not being rolled out to other carers: the actions that the bank took to authorise a second log-in will not be replicated for other customers who desperately need the service.

Of course, I am highlighting what has gone wrong – I am aware there are great examples of things that banks do – but this issue is clearly causing a problem to many carers around the country. I therefore wonder whether the Government might be able to raise the issue with the banks, to ensure that they act responsibly and provide an accessible service to all customers. They should remember that those customers are accessing their own money, and it is their legal right to do so. The practice of not allowing such access is bordering on discrimination

**2nd February 2012: Column 1113**

In not recognising the Equality Act 2010, in accordance with the FOS ruling, carers spend hundreds of pounds going through the legal process of gaining power of attorney, or similar authority. Therefore, it seems illogical that the same legal document permitting access to a person's bank account does not allow access to the service online.

The case that I have raised is not just an isolated incident. Even though Annie has resolved the issue with her bank, she has been told that it was a special allowance for her. She has therefore not stopped campaigning for the facility to be rolled out to other carers in similar situations. I have spent the afternoon with her and her husband. They are a great couple and have fire in their belly when it comes to their campaign – that is a warning shot to the banks, but perhaps also to my hon. friend the Minister. Annie is also a member of the Carers UK Leeds Branch and a governor of the mental health trust, so to say that she knows what she is talking about would be an understatement. As such, she has heard of hundreds of similar cases around the country. Changes to the current practice would have a huge impact on carers and the people they care for. It would be wonderful if a bank took the lead in creating a better system for carers and customers, but I welcome the opportunity to raise this issue in the House today, in the hope that the Government can assist. Carers should not have to spend their valuable spare time, when they are not looking after the people they care for, going through a complex and bureaucratic complaints procedure.

In conclusion, banks should make better provision for carers and take into consideration the needs of their customers. They should therefore ensure that arrangements are in place to assist customers with mental health issues and that staff with specialist knowledge of these requirements are available to assist when necessary. There seem to be a lot of good words coming from the banks, but carers up and down the country are still facing many serious problems. I believe, unless the Minister can tell me otherwise, that what we need is a stronger code of practice to assist carers. It would be most helpful if he would be willing to meet a delegation to discuss this matter. After all, time is precious for all of us these days, but is particularly so for carers.

Exchequer Secretary to the Treasury {Mr. David Gauke}: I should like to begin by thanking my hon. friend the Member for Pudsey [Stuart Andrew] for securing a debate on this issue and for setting out so clearly the circumstances that carers face and the problems that might exist with the banking system. I am also grateful to him for setting out the difficulties that Mr and Mrs Dransfield have faced and telling us of their determination to address them. I sympathise with the difficult circumstances that can be faced by many carers, who make an increasingly important and valuable contribution to our society by supporting those who may be less able, for various reasons, to live an independent life.

The Government are committed to improving access to financial services and, in particular, to bank accounts. It has been amply demonstrated that having a bank account is an essential aspect of modern life for any...

**2nd February 2012: Column 1114**

...individual. My hon. friend set out those circumstances clearly in the context of his constituents. It is clear that many individuals might need the assistance of a carer to help them manage their money, including people with a disability as well as the elderly.

I hope that it will be helpful if I briefly set out the regulations that apply in this area. Banks' and building societies' treatment of their customers is governed by the Financial Services Authority in its banking conduct of business sourcebook. The sourcebook includes a general requirement for firms to provide a prompt, efficient and fair service to all their customers. That includes older people, the disabled, and those who lack capacity to manage their account on their own. In addition, like all service providers, banks and building societies are bound, under the Equalities Act 2010 – which my hon. friend mentioned – to make reasonable adjustments for disabled people in the way they delivery their services. This may include allowing for a carer or deputy to act for the disabled person.

It is of course right that the banks and building societies have put in place measures to protect their customers and themselves from fraud. They clearly need to satisfy themselves of their customers' identity, both for commercial reasons and to meet their obligations under the Money Laundering Regulations

2007. Before a bank or building society can let someone manage the account of another person, it must have proof of the name and address of the account holder and of the person who will have legal responsibility for managing the account. It must also see evidence of that person's authority to control the account holder's money. When a carer has been given formal authority to manage another person's finances through a power of attorney or court order, or by acting as a deputy, this can be proven through official documentation. However, when a person does not lack capacity to take decisions about their affairs but requires assistance to access their account, the situation can be more difficult. I accept that the case described by my hon. friend falls into the former category.

It is worth noting that most banks offer their customers a range of channels through which to access their bank accounts, including by telephone or in a branch. It might well be that channels are better suited to allowing access to a bank account via a deputy carer or other representative. I also note that the British Bankers' Association has provided on its website information on banking for those with less capacity.

I nevertheless agree with my hon. friend that older people, the disabled and their carer should be able to benefit from the convenience of an online service. With online banking, it is even more important that security measures are in place to prevent unauthorised persons from accessing customers' accounts. There is no opportunity for a member of the bank staff to verify the identity of a carer or representative acting on behalf of a customer. Customers have a duty to protect the security details they are given in order to minimise the rise of financial crime. This may preclude sharing their log-in details with the carer.

My hon. friend set out the unique difficulty faced by those who need the assistance of a carer to access their bank account. As with the application of identity checks more generally, there is a balance to be struck between maximising security for customers and facilitating access...

**2nd February 2012: Column 1115**

...for customers who need the help of a carer. The services offered by banks and building societies are evolving all the time, and I would urge the industry to ensure that account is taken of this issue in the development of online services.

I would like to thank my hon. friend the Member for Pudsey once again for bringing this issue to the attention of the House and Government. I have taken note of his comments about the campaign on this issue. I am sure this is not the last we will hear of this matter either from my hon. friends, or indeed from others. I for one – and the Government as a whole – would be interested to hear from individuals facing some of the difficulties from banks and building societies about how, in the course of improving their services, they are approaching the issue of permitting access for those who require the assistance of a carer. Treasury officials will pick up in their discussion with current account providers the very points that my hon. friend has made this evening.

**2nd February 2012: Column 1116**

I am sure that our hon. friend the Financial Secretary, who leads on the matters but is unavailable today, would be delighted to meet my hon. friend, Annie and her husband, and others, as the matter develops, to look at proposals to address this concern. I assure my hon. friend and the House that we will continue to monitor this issue in the context of improving access to banking more generally and in the context of the Government's action to support carers.

I am grateful to my hon. friend for raising this important issue. He has set out clearly and very well the concerns of his constituents. I assure him that his words have been heard clearly by the Treasury, and I am sure they will have been heard clearly by banks and building societies as well. *The document of the debate can be found on Hansard.*

November 2016 Statement of Support to the Minister – Author Val Hewison, Chief Executive Officer, Carers Leeds Val. hewison@carersleeds.org.uk

To whom it may concern,

Carers Leeds is the main carer support service in the city with an aim to ensure appropriate information, advice and support is available to carers to sustain them in their caring role.

We support the issues that are being brought to the Financial Secretary with regard to concerns and barriers carers face when supporting the person they are caring for around banking issues.

Carers Leeds supports many carers who are faced with problems particularly around online banking for the people they care for. It is a crucial issue that affects many people, and we would support banking systems reviewing their policies and procedures to ensure obstacles are removed, whilst maintaining the very important issues of confidentiality and consent.

We believe this can be achieved by open and transparent communication which will lead to a consistent approach by all banks and in consultation with family carers, to bring about change.

By working together, I believe we can improve banking policies which will lead to better experiences, less stress and a more joined-up approach to supporting both family carers and the person they are caring for.

**7th November 2016 – Meeting with the Minister: Re Better Banking for Carers**

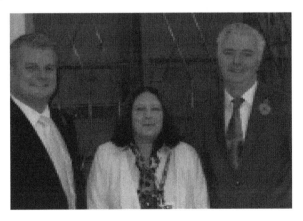

Prior to the meeting with the Minister on this issue I prepared and sent this report him.

Introduction

I am an unpaid carer. Caring for thirty-nine years and still caring.

My banking experience over several years caused considerable distress, anxiety and inconvenience to me and my son. An experience that is not unique amongst the many carers I speak to. To be accused of banking online illegally makes a mockery of the laws in place for a deputy through the Court of Protection and lasting power of attorney. Depositing these legalities to help your loved one is time-consuming and an expensive undertaking, a decision that is not taken lightly but can be undermined instantly by banks in terms of finances.

Managing my son's account using online banking seemed to go well at first, for a year or so, then it all went terribly wrong.

Finally, after several years of going through the complaints procedure, many meetings with my MP Stuart Andrew and the ombudsman in connection with the numerous issues this false accusation had on me, the complaint was upheld in my favour.

My online banking was reinstated. The ombudsman's report stated that the bank's stance is not consistent with general industry practice and suggested that the bank might have broken the law requiring equal treatment for able and disabled customers.

Thousands of carers all over the country have had, or still have, problems with banking for their loved ones online and in branches. We need to recognise and rectify this issue to make

Banking Better for Carers.

Co-production is a way forward in terms of working with the professionals, who have the expertise in banking and finances, meeting with experts in unpaid caring to find a solution. In practice, we should involve people who use services so that they may be included and consulted and that both parties work together from start to completion. How many carers use the services? What are their situations? Definition and discussion is important in order to improve services, products and break down barriers. Organisations can become agents for change as opposed to only being service providers. How can we do this?

In view of this document being presented to the director of the Financial Conduct Authority, the Banking Payment and Policy Team, Public Affairs Team, the British Bankers' Association and Stuart Andrew MP, I would like to take this opportunity to thank you all immensely for your time and support in this matter. I gratefully request that all concerned professionals consider these proposals and recommendations with a view to agreeing a definite action that we can move forward with at the end of this meeting.

**Aims**

To encourage co-production, a meeting of minds in order to instigate and assist to find a shared solution.

To meet with the Financial Conduct Authority, the British Bankers' Association and other appropriate organisations to discuss the barriers carers face when managing their loved ones' finances.

In practice, we should engage with people who use services in terms of them being consulted, included and working together throughout as well as advocate how organisations and their workforce can become instrumental in change as well as being product providers.

Ensure banks give carers the recognition they deserve and see them as experts in the individual financial issues they have to deal with. What systems will and will not work for them.

Discuss and devise a system whereby the business product and service is reshaped to suit the needs of the carer and service user and not the other way round.

Discuss and implement publicity for a 'Carer-Friendly Bank.'

Organise and establish a pilot scheme with carers, services users and professionals.

**Objectives**

Review and develop new and existing methods, policies, systems and procedures in order to fulfil the needs of carers and service users therefore providing them with a stress-free way of banking online and in branches.

**My recommendations**

Commission a bank/s that is/are willing to take the lead in endeavouring to reshape the provision of banking for carers and their loved ones.

Set up a steering group to discuss what needs to be accomplished and how this can be implemented.

Look at and discuss existing branch and online procedures, policies and systems in order to identify the fractures that act as barriers to carers. I was told that online banking was a separate entity from the branches.

Explore and discuss how we can successfully eliminate these barriers in order to make way for a fresh, proactive, constructive and unchallenging method that is carer-friendly.

Develop a database that flags up all carers and service users regardless of whether they hold a legal document or not, to enable staff to identify and understand that their more vulnerable customers and carers will need a little bit more time and help from a professional that knows about these difficulties and complexities.

Devise a Carer-Friendly notification and logo for banks to display.

Devise a card for carers that ties in with database information to prove identification of the holder of a legal document which could include a PIN number for extra security.

The report continues with recommendations for staff training of a carer's situation and needs in addition to improved communication and verbal and visual information.

## Conclusion of Meeting

The Economic Secretary to the Treasury and City Minister Mr Simon Kirby, at the Houses of Parliament, stated that the report and recommendations were valid and important and the action he would take would be to write a letter to the banks on this issue. In addition it was agreed that Stuart Andrew MP would table this question: "What progress has been made on improving access to online and in-branch banking for carers?"

I believe the meeting to have been extremely proactive and positive and concluded with an action I believed could take this issue forward.

**10th July 2018:** A further meeting was held, arranged by my MP, with the FCA (Financial Conduct Authority). At this meeting, I presented my case on Better Banking for Carers, explaining that change was needed to improve banking, with policies, procedures and systems put in place to cater for all carers and service users, emphasising that carers should be involved with the planning processes at all stages. I suggested that a pilot scheme be implemented at local level with a view to future expansion at a national level. In order to achieve this, I suggested the FCA and I should work together, along with other senior staff at various banks, to meet and discuss my proposals and how they could be implemented.

**October 2018:** It was agreed that another meeting be arranged to discuss this further and to invite the British Bankers' Association, now known as UK Finance, with the hope and anticipation that Better Banking for Carers would advance even further with the proposals.

I travelled to London, once again, with my husband. We sat around the solid and very large table, on chairs of the same making, in a very spacious and stately room waiting for representatives of UK Finance to arrive. Eventually, the PA rang them to find out where they were. As she put the phone down, she told us that they were not attending and would not meet with me but, at some point, would meet with my MP. My MP, like me, was not happy about this.

I remember saying, "Well, I'm just a Yorkshire lass from a small village in Leeds, why would they not want to meet with me?"

Our meeting continued and concluded with the FCA talking about a report they had written. If I had a look at this report, there might be some points in it that I had in mine, along with points that I had made and were not in theirs.

I read the report which was three hundred plus pages long. I made notes along the way, most of it being focused on the elderly and not relevant to what I had in my proposal report. I had expressed that the best way to move forward was to meet and discuss the proposals in my report, eliminating or adding what aspects we could or could not take further, with a view to agreeing a plan of action. This was not taken any further.

I decided to go and talk to the manager of the Yorkshire Bank, at the local branch. She was extremely helpful and interested in Better Banking for Carers. I only intended, so as not to take up too much of her time, to leave my report with her to look at and get back to me.

However, she said, "I'll read it now." She then said she would get in touch with the manager of the customer experience team at the Yorkshire Bank's head office. Not only that, she prepared my document so it could be used for presentation slides on PowerPoint, being a bit of a dinosaur in this area, I was very grateful for her expertise.

Further to this meeting, I was contacted by the customer experiences manager from Head Office. We had an initial meeting and, from this, I was contacted by her again. The manager wrote to me and stated that our initial meeting was very insightful and that she too had read the FCA report, although it was focused very much on the elderly. She felt that there were synergies with carers and vulnerable people, and that she had some thoughts on what they could do to improve.

I was invited to give a talk to the wider management team on my experiences as a carer on this issue and my vision for the future in Better Banking for Carers. The talk was well received and, yet again, my being was flooded with hope and anticipation that together we could bring the proposals to fruition. This did not happen, there may have been other reasons as to why we did not meet again, but I suspect that the biggest factor was that the head office was closing, as was the local branch, however Yorkshire Bank still operates.

> **Personal Reflection**: In this case, the ombudsman was consistent, efficient and professional throughout his investigation of my complaint, and my decision on the compensation offered by the bank was one of acceptance via the ombudsman. However, this major concern, in terms of living through this nightmare of unjustness in order to right

the wrongs of this case from a moral and legal entitlement, took immediate precedence.

Compensation did not even enter into the equation, but it did go a little way to helping with expenses that had gone into compiling this case, like cartridges of ink and paper for the printer, sandwiches and coffee on the train going to London and, at this point, I would like to give a massive 'thank you' to Mick Ward and Ian Brooke-Mawson of the Carers Strategy Board who helped me with one of my train tickets for the many trips I made to London.

Their support for carers with Carers Leeds, along with all the other members of the Board, is exceptional and sincere, and this gesture for me as a carer was greatly appreciated and above and beyond their duty.

I had been accused of being fraudulent, of banking online illegally. I was so upset when I was accused of being a fraud that I really thought I was going to be arrested and taken to prison. I was angry, frightened and tearful, thrown into a state of distress marked by confusion.

The bank account we have is a joint account, whereby I had a card and Jay had a card, but mine was taken away from me. The bank stated that my son might get access to the accounts, and yet the bank set online banking up for me.

The Disability Law Service states that: *it is unlawful for service providers to refuse to serve, or to provide a service on worse terms to a person who is disabled or fail to make a reasonable adjustment for a disabled person, disabled meaning mentally or physically.*

My personal opinion is that a bank is a service provider, therefore, it should be adhering to disability law.

## Branches and Online – Do they communicate with each other?

I was extremely upset when, as a lasting power of attorney for my father, I still received emails from the bank saying: "*Hello Edward, Thank you for being a … Bank customer. We would like to hear about your experience with us. With your help, we want to keep improving and become a better bank. We really mean it when we say we are listening. Our survey should only take a few minutes and lets you tell us exactly what you think and we promise to listen.*"

My father was receiving palliative care at the time I received this email. He passed away a few weeks later. I received another email similar to this after his death, and when I told the bank the emails stopped. If, as a bank, you know that someone is a lasting power of attorney or similar, add their name on the front of the message as well, after all, the email is being sent to the attorney, so this should be a big clue that the customer is not able to handle their own financial affairs.

When anyone has taken the time and paid for a legal document to bank on their loved one's behalf, my lived experience makes a mockery of the legal system and courts when having gone through the procedures of taking out a deputyship through the Court of Protection/lasting power of attorney.

Let's just remind ourselves of what the banks say to us:

*"Let us make life easier for you."*

*"Making your views count."*

*"Making banking easier."*

*The Government stated: "We want to see everybody online."*

*"Tell us what you think that can directly influence what we do in the future."*

My answer to this last statement is: I have been trying to do this from February 2010. We are now ten years on from the first day I was stopped banking online. I will leave you to your own analysis about why the banks do not want to work with me and other carers.

**I have put these questions to the bank:**
- What is the difference between branches and online banking?
- Branches and online – do they communicate with each other?
- Has staff training on financial issues such as this been carried out?

**I have raised these issues:**
- Lack of information, and when there is information, there is a lack of clarity
- Lack of communication and organisation skills
- Mixed messages in terms of policies and procedures

**This is how I felt – impact on the carer**

Angry, upset, patronised, humiliated, anxious, distressed, fatigued, vulnerable, disillusioned, perplexed, confused, suspicious, alarmed, threatened, exasperated, frustrated and physically exhausted.

---

**Personal Reflection:** There are many positives in this lived experience in all aspects but, at the same time, there are just as many negatives from the very people who can bring Better Banking for Carers to fruition and ensure that this predicament never happens again.

These issues of banking are in the public domain, the 'Better Banking for Carers' speech is on Hansard in the Houses of Parliament, forever recorded in the history, to remind us of one the injustices of this state of affairs in 21st century.

Which bank will be the first to discuss and implement the recommendations made in my report? Which bank will be the first to talk to carers in a boardroom and not over the counter of a bank?

---

There are over seven million carers in our country, and I have successfully brought these issues into the open that I know many of you have encountered one way or another, but without the cooperation of the professionals who can make Banking Better for Carers happen, who have said they would take my suggestions on board, they however have not included me in any talks they might have had. We need to see practical changes along with a carer-friendly bank logo on display in all banks.

These are the people, organisations and resources I contacted and used in my research, along with those who gave me a great deal of support and encouragement:

Carers Leeds: supported this campaign from the start. Encouraged and listened to me. Is exemplary in all the services it provides to carers.

Carers UK: support from Matt, Gavin, David, Michael, Imelda, Emily, Fern and many more staff who have since left or retired. Campaign was publicised in their magazines and at Carers UK conferences.

University of Leeds – School of Healthcare: Dr Gary Morris, Dr Elaine McNichol and all previous staff present and retired that I worked with.

Leeds and York Partnership Foundation Trust: Chief Executive Officer Chris Butler and all staff.

Dame Philippa Russell: I had the pleasure of meeting Dame Philippa Russell at a carers' conference in Leeds. I contributed to the many experiences that carers conveyed in connection with various issues. Needless to say, mine was on banking. Dame Philippa Russell spoke to me after the conference and was appalled by what had happened. From then on, she offered her support and we emailed regularly. As a carer herself, she knew only too well the kinds of pressures carers are under and the barriers they face. We corresponded by email and she never ever left one of my emails or calls unanswered.

Leeds City Council: Bridget McGuire, Mick Ward, Ian Brooke-

Mawson and all senior members from various organisations who sat on the Carers Strategy Board.

Councillor Lucinda Yeadon, Leeds City Council: who wrote to the Office of the Public Guardian, Royal Bank of Scotland, HSBC, FSA, Halifax, Lloyds and TSB.

British Bankers' Association: who stated that: *"...we will be using this experience as a case study and will look into the matter further."* Yet were absent from the meeting. The British Bankers' Association was a trade association for the UK banking and financial services sector. From the 1st July 2017 it was merged into UK Finance.

Barclays: who stated in their reply that: *"...there will be no issue with anyone appointed as deputy under a Court of Protection order to be allowed internet access to online banking after the prescribed process for registering."*

Mind: to tell them about the issues, but unfortunately I did not receive a reply.

I called into HSBC to ask about online banking. They rang me back the following day to say: *"You can bank online with us, but it would have to be in Jay's name."* – They said that more discussion was needed on the issue as they were not sure about all their online banking needs.

I contacted the FSA by telephone to ask whether there was a document on guidelines and regulations for online banking for the banks and if there was, was the same document available for customers using online banking? Their answer was: *"No, banks and building societies have their own policies."*

Unless I missed something, I could not find any banking policies when I researched on the internet.

I contacted a local Labour candidate, but did not get a response.

Online banking legislation

Halifax senior staff online banking team banking investigation and their findings

*Money Made Clear: FSA*

*British Bankers' Association: Banking for people who lack capacity*

Transition Information Network

Which? Reviews – Online banking for people who lack capacity

Cash Questions – Banking Online

Caring for someone FSA Money Made Clear – guides

Direct Gov – Disabled people's rights in everyday life

Disability Discrimination Acts

Royal Bank of Scotland, Legal Information

At an event I attended with Time to Change, Lloyds Bank took the 'Time to change pledge'. I had an envelope ready with all the details in of my 'Better Banking for Carers' campaign in the hope I could pass this on to one of the staff. I spoke to one of the senior management in attendance. He listened, as I explained briefly about my experience that was still ongoing and stressed the importance of the pledge 'Time to Change' not just in regard to the stigma of mental health but also in the practical sense of finance as well. He took my document, which also contained recommendations of what banks could do to help carers in these situations. Was I expecting an answer? Yes, I was, even just out of courtesy. I had no answer at all.

Mental Health Foundation – Personal banking. All information relating to banking for carers and service users

Alzheimer's Society and various other mental health charities

**There's a Frog in the Basement: Under The Desk** I was just about to walk into the supermarket, when a lady pushing a wheelchair was on her way out. She stopped me to ask if I would be good enough to look after her mother for a few minutes, whilst she went to the entrance of the car park to wait for the ambulance to arrive so she could direct them to where her mother was. Of course I said I would. Her mother had been taken ill in the supermarket and her daughter, Iris, was on her own. The ambulance soon arrived and, whilst the paramedics got her mother into the ambulance, Iris and I talked a little about caring. She told me that the bank they used had phoned to say that they needed her mother to sign some forms and would she bring her mother into the branch. She explained that it would be very difficult to do so and told them that her mother suffered with Parkinson's disease and dementia.

Parkinson's disease is a complex condition that affects people in different ways with some of the symptoms being tremors, shaking, impaired posture and balance. Balance or postural instability is a tendency to be unstable when standing and affects the reflexes that are essential for maintaining an upright position.

Individuals with disabilities may have difficulty with communication in terms of speech and writing. These are called motor symptoms. Non-motor symptoms that a person may experience are pain and depression.

Iris asked the bank if she could collect the forms from the bank and take them home for her mother to sign and then she would bring them back.

"No," said the bank, "she will have to come in and sign them."

Suffering with a bad leg at the time, and could hardly walk properly herself, Iris took her mother to the bank as requested.

As anyone would be in that situation, Iris was annoyed about this whole business, as she was in her middle sixties and not in good health.

However, Iris limped through the building to the interview room where upon the staff member said, "Oh dear, you don't look to be having a good day."

To which the much stressed daughter replied, "This is an ordinary day for me, love."

Once in the interview room, Iris's mother started to shake considerably, this went unnoticed by the member of staff, until suddenly, Iris's mother slipped out of the wheelchair and landed on the floor underneath the member of staff's desk.

"Now do you understand why I did not want to bring my mother to the bank, she is just not well enough?"

**What Now?**: *The following is an article by an unknown author but was reported in the* Irish Times *– no date available.*

A lady died and the bank billed her for their annual service charges on her credit card and then added late fees and interest on the monthly charge. The balance that had been £0.00 now was somewhere around £60.00. A family member made the telephone call to the bank which went like this:

Family Member: I am calling to tell you that she died in January.

Bank: The account was never closed and the late fees and changes still apply.

Family Member: Maybe you should pass it over to collections.

Bank: Since it is two months past due, it already has been.

Family Member: So, what will they do when they find out she is dead?

Bank: Either report her account to the frauds division or report her to the credit department, maybe both.

Family Member: Do you think God will be mad at her?

Bank: Excuse me?

Family Member: Did you just get what I was telling you... the part about her being dead?

Bank: Sir, you'll have to speak to my supervisor.

*Supervisor comes to the phone.*

Family Member: I'm calling to tell you she died in January.

Bank: The account was never closed and the late fees and charges still apply.

Family Member: You mean you want to collect from her estate?

Bank: [Stammering] Are you her lawyer?

Family Member: No, I am her great-nephew. [Lawyer information given.]

Bank: Could you fax us a certificate of death?

Family Member: Yes, of course.

*[Fax number is given.]*

After receiving the fax.

Bank: Our system just isn't set up for death. I don't know what more I can do to help.

Family Member: Well, if you figure it out that's great, if not, you could just keep billing her. I don't think she will care.

Bank: Well, the late fees and charges do still apply.

Family Member: Would you like her new billing address?

Bank: That might help.

Family Member: Whistdown Cemetery. WI28 OHNO. Plot 106.

Bank: But that is a cemetery, sir!

Family Member: Well, what the ******** do you do with dead people on your planet?

*"Our greatest weakness lies in giving up. The most certain way to succeed is always to try just once more."* – Thomas Edison

**What Now?:** My phone rang.

"Hello Jay."

"Mum?"

"Yes, what's up?"

"Did you say you had put £10 in my account today?"

"Yes, I did. The balance is £10.59."

"I'm with Alice at the shopping centre, and I've tried three cash machines, one said they didn't have any tens, one said it had no money in, and the other wasn't working."

"Just a minute, while I run upstairs to check your accounts on the computer." I logged into the online banking account, at least I could do that now without a problem. "Hold on a minute while I put the details in, and I'll put you another £10 in, and don't forget this has to go back into your savings, because you have used all your benefits for the fortnight in one week."

"Yes, okay Mum."

# CHAPTER 8

# A Vision of Life and Caring in 2050

My name is Marina Gold, and I am connected to Blaze, we live with our children Cell and Echo. My mother, Ember, and my father, Harlin Luna, live with us in one of the levels of our dwelling that has been specifically designed to be self-contained allowing some form of independence, along with peace and quiet, in their elderly and infirm years.

We live in the city of Silvermage which is one of the smaller cities in England; it is clean and spacious, even though they are tall, technology-smart buildings that incorporate natural elements, along with spaces that can be transformed to meet business needs or home living. They stand neatly spaced amongst a landscape of green, rainwater cleansing and absorbent gardens, punctuated with narrow inlets of rainwater channels. The city provides an all-white-and-black, impressive, high-profile, rail transport, using distinguished technology in the form of regional rail stations that run smoothly, quietly, efficiently and speedily to one's favoured destination.

Some of the underground buildings incorporate a series of small, rectangular windows on the surface giving out an illuminated, violet glow visible from the frontage, producing a stunning, atmospheric ambience, yet their main purpose is to serve the green streets of Silvermage with an environmentally friendly water filtration and monitoring network.

Shopping malls of thirty years ago are non-existent, however, in our small city we have a Smart High Technology Centre where holographic fashion shows take place, human robotics and Al shop assistants, who know immediately a client's interests and tastes, are there to help.

The metallic, iridescent, holographic, all-in-one smart suit I am wearing now highlights a clean, subtle, dappled and delicate mix of purple, pinks, silver and blues depicting a warmth and coolness all at the same time, in addition to changing in different lights. I purchased my attire from one of the holographic fashion shows, and of course I had to get the holograph boots to match.

I can change the colour and design of any of my garments via a touch on my smartphone, and most of the sustainable and digital garments have built-in sensors that allow broadcasting data to Cloud, Firebolt or Whirlwind.

We can try on clothes in virtual reality changing rooms and, once decided on, my purchase it will be waiting for me when I get back, delivered into my garden by a flying robot. This is the world we live in, surrounded by artificial intelligence, sustainable and organic materials for clothing and adaptable, wearable technology.

The private residences in my neighbourhood are called Decagons, taken from the original shape's name, which is flat and has ten straight sides, moulded and constructed from recycled plastic. Each of these huge, deep, flat shapes is joined together by thick columns of the same material, horizontally and diagonally, with built-in concourses allowing us a continuous flow of access to all rooms on two, sometimes three or four, levels.

Space-age, state-of-the-art windows complement the design by being installed in each Decagon, allowing views, from all angles, on to our gardens that completely surround our private dwellings with many of them having water features, in addition to the widescreen views of Glass Apple, the innovative, neighbouring urban village a few miles away. In this village, people live in cyclopean, trailblazing hubs and pods with many of them having hydroponic technology for farms, a community that has sustainable energy along with small-scale farming.

We communicate using nothing but our thoughts, by way of collective A1 consciousness that is part of the very fabric of our human brain and can reveal what anyone is thinking. Articles depicting history from the twenty-first century 2016-2018 on communication stated that humanity will abandon speech and communicate through a collective A1 consciousness using nothing but thoughts by 2050, which we are in now. The A1 system is called the hybrid biometric avatar (HIBA).

History also states that in 2008, theoretical physicist, Stephen Hawking, used an infrared switch, mounted on his glasses, which captured the slightest twitch of his cheek, or even direct brain activity [*Google*], which he used to control a cursor or select words on his speech device.

Several groups of neuroscientists around the world, at that time, were working to develop a more intuitive way to communicate by converting the brain signals of what users would like to say into sound using a voice synthesiser, thereby turning thoughts into words.

One of the quotes I saw, from a politician called Matt Hancock, made at the time of a horrendous pandemic in 2020 called the coronavirus, Covid-19, in which he stated that patients wouldn't go back from online GP consultations after the pandemic, adding that they must not lose the digital advances that had been made during the Covid-19 crisis. Since that statement was made, all those years ago, we have advanced astronomically and, in order to tell you about the way I live, I am communicating my thoughts into a virtual communication system which will transfer my thoughts into words for the sole use of this 'think piece'.

Blaze and I each have a form of transport which is the length of a six-seater, private jet. This ultimate mode of transference is engineered to make a vertical take-off, and landing, along with being extremely powerful and fast-moving. In addition to having a palatial interior, the extreme and exposed materials are of a high-calibre colour, mine is a chromatic black and white whilst Blade's is the same but in silver. To operate our Airland transference, we input our navigation and destination data into a sophisticated interface which works on the highest possible speed, called warp speed. Once this action is completed, we are ready to soar through the specifically designed skyways.

In this year of 2050, our children Cell and Echo do not go to what was called a school in 2020. History books tell me that children went to a building called a school every day, where they sat on chairs in front of desks ready for a lesson to begin by the teacher. Although schools and universities are still in existence, they are designed with collaborative spaces and online platforms, mainly used for specific types of learning. Most learning for children is done by way of e-learning, i-learning platforms, mobile video learning and courses which are driven by interest and passion and not mainly by a degree.

We do not use what was once called money in Silvermage, but instead it is called electronic cash, this is money but is identified as a non-specific value which has been replaced by credits for specific future goods and services. The type of money we hold in bank accounts, what are currently money transactions, will be replaced by networked barter of these credits.

The lines of engagement for people in our chamber are varied; Blade is a data detective, whilst I enjoy the role of a digital rehabilitation counsellor. Cell is already researching what it takes for him to be an extinct species revivalist whilst Echo wants to pursue her passion and interest in becoming a virtual reality actress.

To give us all the nutrients, sustenance and energy we require, we consume caplets that come in a vast amount of different tastes and are immensely satisfying. We are led to believe that the caplets we consume are just as fulfilling and enjoyable as a full, three-course meal would have been in 2020. Oh my Trojan, to even think that I would be faced with one of these three-course meals on a platter. We just decide which kind of caplet we want and enjoy, I am so glad that I do not have to come into contact with what was called 'dirty dishes' in the 2020s. It seems that humans, in those days, did not have a great deal of time to themselves, as they actually had to shop for food, prepare it and cook it, this method to us is an antediluvian way for victualling.

Although my parents, Ember and Harlin, live with us, they are part of the wider spectrum of the 'Lifework of Care' in our city. They have their own level within our Decagon; I believe this would have been called an annexe many years ago.

A humanoid solution specifically designed for the care of the elderly is called a Carebot. The Carebot is equipped with state-of-the-art navigation, sensory and perception systems that allows them to complete tasks like picking up a remote aid or retrieving a Medican canister, in addition to taking temperatures and vital signs using facial recognition. Our friendly Carebot assists my parents with all personal care, such as cleaning oneself and feeding. Some of our more bedridden elderly have a Robobear that can lift you from one place to another, along with any other physical assistance that is required.

One of the medicines in use is nano medicine; the definition of this refers to natural, incidental or manufactured material comprising particles either in an unbound state or as an aggregate. Nano medicine is an artificial intelligence equipped with algorithms which will relieve emergency room personnel of tending to large numbers of walk-in patients. These nano materials are used for diagnoses, monitoring control, prevention and treatment of diseases.

I have conveyed to you many aspects of our lives and lifestyle in Silvermage which are incredibly different to the lives of people in various cities in 2020. The atmosphere is clean and fresh, as is our land. We do not have the many difficulties that faced society in 2020 like waste and litter, violence and crime, pollution, cruelty and prejudice, whereas respect, pride, courtesy, compassion, and many more moral and social values, demonstrated by a good deal of the population in 2020, are now the most predominant and powerful traits in our world.

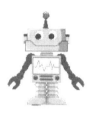

## A Vision of Life and Caring in 2050

## Facts, Figures, Research and Predictions

The passage that follows depicts various beliefs and perceptions of what the world could be like in 2050. Some of the advanced technology we are already seeing and using, and advances in all aspects of life, are most likely to start with conducting research. This research is undertaken by way of collection of data, documentation, critical information, analysis and interpretation.

Theoretical assumptions are made, conceptual ideas and thoughts explored, along with research design, interpretation and invention, which invariably combines summaries, conclusions and recommendations.

Opinions and views are shared between the experts in a particular subject that can take the form of critical analysis, denial, agreement or disagreement, refusal and constructive criticisms, all of which may contribute to revolutionary and groundbreaking inventions intended for the greater good of society. This particular chapter took me, in terms of research, to a futuristic world that I tried hard to imagine myself living in. Some of what I have described in Marina's world is exciting, some of it scary and unbelievable, and a part of it which is happening today. Predictions can be disconcerting and unsettling, whilst others are favourable, thoughts and reasonings are highlighted, so I leave it to you to devise your own theory, opinion and decision on this theme.

**Population and Dementia** Research suggests that in 2050 the world's population aged sixty years and older will be two billion, up from nine hundred million from 2015. The number of people in the UK living with dementia is stated to be 850,00, with one in six people over the age of eighty with dementia, and this number is predicted to rise to over two million by 2050 as the population ages.

One is six people will be over the age of sixty-five for the first time ever in 2050 and will outnumber children under the age of five.

**A Future City** that will see underground farming, a city that is fully accessible to the disabled, with unfettered access to goods and services in addition to lighter and cheaper bladeless wind turbines situated on the rooftops of buildings providing supplementary energy, along with drones for commuting, which it is predicted, will be powerful and large enough to transport people within cities.

**Nursing Homes** Tokyo's Shin-tomi nursing home is probably one of the most high-tech nursing homes in the world. Residents interact with around twenty different types of robots designed to assist with care, comfort and loneliness. Rudimentary conversations befriend the elderly along with helping them to make and receive video calls, monitor blood pressure, heart rate, respiration and sleeping state, they can call emergency services, offer exercise guidance, daily health briefings and play music to reduce stress. [*Hack and Craft*]

Research predicts some of the more unpleasant and unacceptable situations, that could arise, being: poorer air pollution, populations that might not have adequate water, the number of people living in cities tripling, hurricanes might become more frequent, and large-scale blackouts may become commonplace, in addition to the increase of cyberattacks, fish stocks could be overexploited, or fully exploited, and lack of proper nutrition could affect children acutely stunting development. The more positive side of the predictions are that: child mortality rates will be lower, vaccines and cures for many diseases will be found, a better understanding of the process behind Alzheimer's will lead experts closer to a cure. Humans could live forever as computerised brains, and there will be no more poor countries, in addition to the assumption that we will have the ability to rely almost exclusively on renewable, clean energy.

**Summary**

Whatever or wherever the future takes us in the next thirty years, particularly in caring, we must not forget the most fundamental factor of mankind concerning our loved one's care and the humanity we demonstrate.

Innovation, medicine and science, without question, have their place in our world, and they have given us many life-saving resources. But behind each and every one of these exceptional brains is a person, or team, that has put their life, soul and passion into making one's life better, and it is exactly this, the human brain, the human heart, soul and compassion, that I doubt no one can replicate in a machine, that no robot in thirty years' time will have, because it is very difficult to comprehend, at this point in time, how this will be achieved.

At a conference I attended on mental health, one of the attendees, a carer, brought up the subject of drug and alcohol addiction. They stated that many carers are also dealing with these problems that their loved ones have as well other mental health issues, yet these carers seem to be forgotten. From observing the body language of others, it was obvious that some of the other attendees felt uncomfortable talking about this particular aspect of caring. This seems to be the dark side of caring, and some people even mock or laugh this aspect away, but I can assure you that there is nothing funny about addiction, as many carers have to deal with the impact of it on their loved ones and their families because, for them, there is no light relief, there is no respite.

I hope that, in some small way, my many experiences have helped in an empathic way, that historically lessons can be learned for the future, that carers, universally, will be taken more seriously and that new carers will be forewarned and forearmed about the pitfalls that occur and, last but not least, organisations that can help carers more will do so.

I leave you with my philosophy which is try to be proactive, positive, organised, prepared, focused and strong. Thank you for being my fellow carers, and I hope you have a lot fun with the activities and interesting debates with the issues depicted.

Contact: Annie

# CHAPTER 9

# Activities

## Activity 1

### The Perceptual Table

Perception: The ability to interpret or become aware of something through the senses.

Practical: Being aware of a situation, identifying and perceiving actions to take

Discuss the possible consequences of a person's action or words

(overleaf)

## Perceptual Table

Use this table to identify the factors of the emotional, physical, social, spiritual, and psychological impact, in any of the experiences depicted, has had on the carer and service user.

| | | | | |
|---|---|---|---|---|
| **EMOTIONAL** | Anxious about potential outcomes | Naïve about what I do in certain situations | Worried about my loved one's future<br><br>Relationship with partner breaking down | No colleagues<br><br>No friends |
| **PHYSICAL/ PRACTICAL** | What help can I get for my mental health? | Trying to take in all that has been said to me by professionals | What help can I get for my physical health? | The impact on finances when a carer stops work to care full-time |
| **SOCIAL** | Time-consuming tasks: phone calls, letters, conversations, instructions | Very little time for leisure or to relax | Not many friends left | |
| **SPIRITUAL** | No real understanding, empathy or compassion from some people | If one has a religious faith it can be easily lost | I have faith in the medical professionals in whatever aspect, that they are there to help us, then it all goes wrong | |
| **PSYCHO-LOGICAL** | Stress<br><br>Mind overloading<br><br>Depression | | | |

| Worrying about where to go for help when needed with lots of issues | Thinking of the questions I need to ask in a certain situation | Very troubled over my loved one's illness | Frustrated at not being able to look after myself properly. Lack of time and finances, several of the reasons | Angry, Upset, Belittled, Humiliated, Vulnerable, Disillusioned, Perplexed, Alarmed, Confused, Suspicious, Distressed |
|---|---|---|---|---|
| Difficulty in eating, sleeping and concentrating for worrying about all the things I have to do | Feeling exhausted all the time | Stress can have an impact on physical health | | |
| | | | | |
| I have faith in external agencies but then this is lost because of a lack of understanding on what the carer has to deal with and because of their own procedures and policies | | | | |
| | | | | |

Blank one for leaders to print out

| | | | | |
|---|---|---|---|---|
| **EMOTIONAL** | | | | |
| **PHYSICAL/ PRACTICAL** | | | | |
| **SOCIAL** | | | | |
| **SPIRITUAL** | | | | |
| **PSYCHO- LOGICAL** | | | | |

# Activity 2

# Moral Values, Social Skills and Communication

## How good are your communication skills?

**ORAL COMMUNICATION SKILLS**

☐ Do you support the carer by giving information, suggestions, options and ideas?

☐ Do you make requests and constructive criticisms with clarity and tact?

☐ Do you speak clearly and audibly, using appropriate volume, pace, pitch and intonation?

☐ Do you select an appropriate level of formality?

☐ Do you structure your talk that demonstrates awareness of listeners?

☐ Do you have the ability to paraphrase or summarise?

☐ Do you share information, opinions and ideas?

☐ Do you seek information, opinions and ideas from others?

☐ Do you build on and support ideas and points made by others?

☐ Do you demonstrate compromise? What other solutions do you find to reconcile differences with clients and colleagues?

☐ Do you evaluate the strengths and weaknesses of your clients and colleagues?

☐ Do you demonstrate the ability to summarise the substance and direction of the group and in a one-to-one client discussion?

We do not know what a person's moral values and social skills are like until we get to know them, which is why I describe them as unseen. However, they are values and skills that are an integral part of training, communication and caring.

**YOUR OWN EVALUATION: COMMENTS ON YOUR ORAL COMMUNICATION SKILLS**

## Activity 3

## Who's Knocking on my Door?

## Mantle of the Expert (MoE)

Involves the creation of a fictional world where students assume the roles of experts in a designated field. A problem or task is established and the students are contracted in or framed as an enterprise – a team of experts using imaginative role play to explore issues.

Mantle of the Expert was developed by Dorothy Heathcote at Newcastle University in the 1970s/80s. An internationally renowned authority on drama for learning, Heathcote's aim was to provide non-drama specialists with an approach that would support them in using drama across the curriculum. She believed that drama was an underused approach outside drama studios and could be used as a powerful medium for learning across the curriculum. [*Wikipedia*]

I had the privilege of attending one of her three-day training courses at the Newman College of Higher Education in Birmingham, now a university.

**Key points:**

- Mantel of the Expert: Being oneself but looking at the situation through special eyes.
- Role Playing: Being in a role representing an attitude or point of view.
- Characterising: Representing an individual lifestyle which is somewhat markedly different from the student's own.
- Acting: Selecting symbol, movements, gesture and voice to represent a particular individual to others. Acting can be in the form of presenting or performing.

**"I don't know who you are until I get to know you"**

- Moral values are: ideas and principles that guide people on how to behave.
- Social skills are: what we use to communicate and interact with each other, verbally and non-verbally, through gestures, body language and personal appearance.
- How important are moral and social skills to us all?
- Unseen values are: traits like honesty, punctuality, compassion and integrity, loyalty, patience, fairness, kindness with negative ones being unkindness, unforgiving, uncaring.
- How do you demonstrate to carers and service users that you have decent moral values and social skills?
- How do you adapt your skills in different situations?

## Conversations

Have some fun and start a conversation with any of the following of your choice.

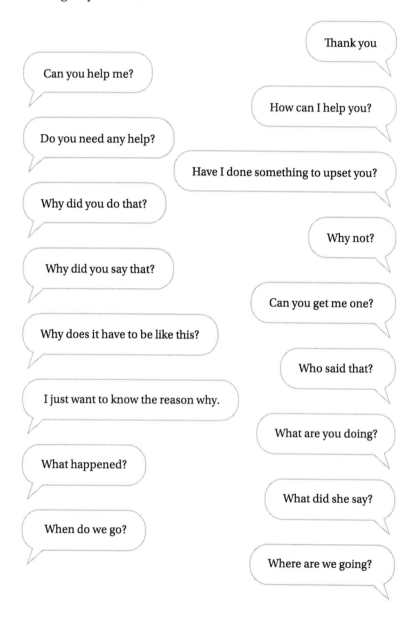

Thank you

Can you help me?

How can I help you?

Do you need any help?

Have I done something to upset you?

Why did you do that?

Why not?

Why did you say that?

Can you get me one?

Why does it have to be like this?

Who said that?

I just want to know the reason why.

What are you doing?

What happened?

What did she say?

When do we go?

Where are we going?

## Activity 4

## Role Play

**Role play** is not acting; it is about putting yourself in another's person shoes, in other people's situations, in order to understand their different emotions in various situations and what it is like in a variety of circumstances.

Role Play:
- Offers insights into the feelings and attitudes of others
- Looks at the problems and human behaviour of relationships
- Problems, issues or circumstances are often perceived from a new or novel point of view
- Encourages a more active participation other than discussion
- Extends what may be detailed, intellectual discussion into the realms of emotional experience

## Role play is not acting; it is about:

- Defining a problem and establishing a situation/resolution using the above qualities and skills.
- Deciding on each person's character and its role, for example a student, a professional, or any other character you think appropriate.

## Role Play Activity

- From the speech bubbles below devise a scene and role play it
- Discuss and analyse what was said and how it was said
- Discuss the use of words
- Discuss body language and eye contact
- Repeat the exercise turning any negative statements and the tone in which they were spoken into positive ones.
- Devise your own situations and circumstances to go with dialogue
- Devise your own dialogue to make new scenarios
- Demonstrate your scenario

Said to a carer by a professional. Why are you asking me that?

Why did you tell me it had been sorted out, when it clearly has not?

I cannot discuss this issue with you over the phone.

If you miss your hospital appointment three times you are struck off. Basically it's three strikes and you're out. That is just the way it is.

Is he with you? Sorry, I can't discuss this unless he is with you.

She's not in today; I'll get her to call you back next week. Sorry, No there is no one to cover her or check her emails, it's a case of waiting till she is back in the office.

Said to a carer whose dad has Alzheimer's and needs his daughter with him. You can't go in there with him.

Said to carer in a mental health hospital, by a professional, when she was in his room helping him get settled, after just being admitted. Get out.

Give that to me.

You go.

I'm sorry, but you are not the patient.

I'll take that

He's off sick.

You will have to do that.

Just wait here.

You'll have to go somewhere else; we do not do that here.

You'll just have to keep ringing to see if we have any appointments.

She's on leave.

There's no one here at the moment.

## Activity 5a

### Now That's What I Call Care Share

I'M SO BUSY MY HEAD IS PINGING
*Discussion Points*

**POWER**

FULL OF ENERGY OR
RUNNING ON FUMES?

**ON**

HOW DO YOU GET STARTED
ON A MORNING?

Are you in control of the circumstances
and your responsibilities?

**PLAY**

IN YOUR CARING ROLE,
WHAT ARE YOU DOING TODAY?

IN YOUR FAMILY LIFE,
WHAT ARE YOU DOING TODAY?

HOW DO YOU ORGANISE YOUR DAY?

**VOLUME**

WHAT IS THE VOLUME
OF YOUR WORKLOAD?

DO YOU PRIORITISE?

DID YOU GET SOME
PEACE AND QUIET TODAY?

TRACKS

DID YOU FULLY COMPLETE A TASK,
IF NOT WHY NOT?

THERE'S A FROG IN THE BASEMENT...
....WHAT NOW?

HOW MANY INTERRUPTIONS HAVE YOU
HAD TO DEAL WITH TODAY THAT ARE
NOT PART OF YOUR NORMAL ROUTINE?

DO YOU FLIT FROM ONE JOB TO ANOTHER
OR SKIP THEM ALTOGETHER?

SKIP

What are your coping mechanisms?

MIXED MESSAGES

MIXER

DID YOU HAVE TIME TO PAUSE
FOR A THOUGHT?

PAUSE FOR PLANNING?

PAUSE

PAUSE FOR REFLECTION?
PAUSE FOR ASSESSMENT?

GROOVES

ARE YOU STUCK WITH A PROBLEM,
IS THERE A FAULT?

ARE YOU TIRED/POORLY?

HAS YOUR MIND HAD A POWER SURGE
OR A POWER CUT?

REPEAT
PLAY

ARE YOU GOING AROUND IN CIRCLES
AND FIND YOURSELF BACK
AT SQUARE ONE?

ARE YOU BOUNCING
FROM TRACK TO TRACK?

SPINNING

TOO MUCH TO DO,
HOW DO YOU STOP?

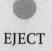

EJECT

NOT AN OPTION/AN IMPOSSIBILITY

OFF

HOW DO YOU SWITCH OFF?

**Activity 5b**

**Care Share – Let's Keep a Sense of Humour**

- Devise a title for a song in connection with anything to do with caring.
- You can adapt existing song titles and artists' names.
- Alternatively, you can devise a completely new one.
- If you wish, you can even devise the full lyrics to go with the title.

Below are some examples of made-up ones and original song titles. Let us keep laughter in our lives.

- 'Problems Keep Falling On My Head'
- 'You Keep Me Hangin' On' – Aretha Franklin
- 'All You Need Is Patience'
- 'Take Control Of Your Actions'
- 'Don't Worry, Be Happy' – Bobby McFerrin
- 'Out Of The Blue' – Debbie Gibson
- 'Everyday Things'
- 'I'm Going Round In Circles'
- 'Wannabe' – Spice Girls: You know what I want what I really, really want; I wanna... – put your own words in.
- 'What's The Worst Thing That Could Happen?'
- 'Oh What A Night' – The Dells
- 'What Am I Doing Now?'
- 'Why Did I Just Say That?'
- 'Something's Burning' – Kenny Rogers
- 'I Just Hit My Head On Another Brick Wall'
- 'What Is It Now?'
- 'Our House' – Madness
- 'Let's Hear It For The Carers'

- 'There Is No One In The Office But The Answerphone Is On...'
- 'Things Can Only Get Better' – Howard Jones
- 'When The Going Gets Tough' – Billy Ocean
- 'Walk Of Life' – Dire Straits
- 'Why Do You Do This To Me?'
- 'Even The Bad Times Are Good' – The Tremeloes

**Activity 6**

**Talk About Words**

**Words related to the Lived Experiences for you to consider and discuss**

From you own experiences, in your personal or professional life, choose a word from the list below that is related to it. Say why you chose it and in what kind of scenario it was used.

- Choose a word that reminds you of a situation you have been in.
- Choose a word that reminds you of a problem you have had to deal with.
- Choose a word that that has led you to think more about challenging, questioning, and policies and procedures.
- Choose a word that reminds you of any situation you have been in where you felt there had been a lack of communication or miscommunication.
- Choose a word that you feel has connections with anger. How do you deal with this emotion?
- Choose a word that is associated with being upset, isolated or unsupported.
- Give an example of good and poor verbal communication.

- Problems issues
- Difficulties
- Surprise
- Shock
- Procedures
- Policies

- Attitudes
- Communication
- Body language
- Terminology
- Challenges
- Barriers

- Injustices
- Feelings
- Emotions
- Moral skills
- Social skills
- Systems
- Protocol
- Image
- Presentation
- Language
- Appropriate
- Inappropriate
- Derogatory
- Vulnerable
- Good practice
- Thoughts
- Beliefs
- Complexities
- History
- Background
- Future
- Vision
- Practical
- Change
- Social change
- Carers' rights
- What's gone wrong?
- How can we improve?
- Hospitals
- Inpatients
- Day centres
- Outpatients

- Alzheimer's
- Carers assessments
- Funded nursing care
- Hospital assessments
- Continuing care treatment
- Initiative
- Proactive
- Positive
- Negative
- Confidence
- Knowledge
- Understanding
- Empathy
- Compassion
- Love
- Attention
- Kindness
- Sensitivity
- Ignorance
- Listening skills
- Common sense
- Logic
- Respect
- Dignity
- Observation
- Frustration
- Disillusioned
- Mental health
- Physical health
- Punctuality
- Honesty

- Clarity
- Transparency
- Care homes
- Support
- Understanding
- Exhaustion

- Depression
- Medication
- community care
- GPs
- Achievements
- Trust

## Activity 7

## Talk, Listen, Respond

## Communication

Aim: To practice effective communication

This is important in professional and daily life because effective communication builds a better relationship, prevents problems, creates a good working relationship and can help you achieve your goals.

Read the following tips before you embark on the following activity:

- Effective listening. Really listen and show interest to what is being said to you.
- Listen to yourself when you are speaking to others.
- Try to give positive and constructive replies.
- Constructive criticism is useful, critical and cynical criticism is not.
- Be aware of the tone of your voice.
- Keep a calm voice when dealing with a difficult issue.
- Be aware of your body language.
- Speak slowly, clearly and with clarity. You will lose the interest of others if you speak too quickly or mumble.
- Keep an open mind in all aspects of conversation.
- Think about solutions, options or compromise to the issue.
- In a difficult situation agree to listen to each other and agree to disagree amicably.
- Don't interrupt.
- Verbal communication i.e. face to face, telephone. Written

communication i.e. letters, emails.
* Non-verbal communication – body language i.e. eye contact, gestures.
* Think about fluency of speech, tone, pace, pitch and intonation.
* If you do not understand something that has been said, always ask.

## Start a conversation from one of the sentences below

* Have we been here before?
* He said to wait here for him.
* We might as well give up and go home.
* You don't have to stay if you don't want to.
* He won't confess anything now.
* Don't you have any self-respect?
* When did you get here?
* How did you get in here?
* How did you do that?
* How can I make you believe me?
* Where is the money now?
* You have no idea what I have been through today.
* I have never seen anything like it in my life.
* Why did you do that?

## My Mantle

*We have a great deal of responsibility, and we play a vital role in terms of holding an extremely important position and saving the government billions of pounds.*

Many carers deal with every single aspect of the service user's life. I have found making a list of all the things I do for my loved one on a daily basis really helps, and then include weekly and monthly tasks. Again, as I said previously, these lists are useful when having to fill in forms like the Personal Independence Payment (PIP) or to convey to professionals verbally what you do as a carer and what help you need. Keep your list up to date by adding or deleting as appropriate.

Many carers have to take responsibility for some, or all, of the following:
- Bankers
- Budget holders
- Primary auditors
- Letter writers for appeals, tribunals, complaints
- Meetings to attend in connection with your loved one's care
- Care support at home/agencies
- Care home
- Doctors' appointments
- Hospital appointments
- Dental appointments
- Outpatient appointments
- Community mental health
- Community psychiatric nurse
- District nurses
- Medication

- Chiropody
- Hairdressers
- Social worker
- Reviews
- Assessments
- Day centres
- Audits direct payments – social services
- Deputy through the Court of Protection, power of attorney
- Deferred payments
- Cost of care
- Laundry
- Cook
- Cleaner
- Shopping
- Hygiene needs
- Bank cards
- Benefits

And don't forget 'there's a frog in the basement' as well. That is when you have to drop everything in order to deal with a minor or major matter. It's just that you have to think on your feet of the best way to deal with the incident. Keep a note of all these incidents, as these are also useful when asked by professional bodies for further details of your loved one's care.

Issues that sometimes arise that affect your loved one because:
- a person is unreliable
- care worker is absent – no replacement today
- incident
- accidental
- information, verbal or written, is misleading/misguided/ inaccurate/invalid

- household appliances can be faulty and/or break down
- keys are lost/stolen
- bank cards are lost/stolen
- bus passes lost/stolen
- in an emergency if your loved one needs money if they can't get home, have you got a proactive plan ready?
- systems, policies and procedures change – and you didn't know about it

From a pint of milk that is needed urgently, a fridge that's been unplugged accidentally, to a major gas leak in the road and your loved one is evacuated for two days and nights, how do you stay calm? What do you do?

This actually happened to my son. He came to stay with us and, at that point, the milk did not matter, as we had some to make a cuppa. Under these circumstances, when people are at risk, the company will get accommodation for you in a local, well-known place that guarantees a good night's sleep or similar if they have not got relatives/friends to go to. When the problem has been rectified, and your loved one can go back to their home, get the milk on the way back. Just hope they have some teabags left in the cupboard!

**Your own Health and Well-being: How are you managing Caring and Work?**

If you are facing difficulties at work, due to caring, speak to your employer, seek advice and support and, as always, make your own personal notes – I know keep going on about this, but it really helps, as you may need that information later.

As the saying goes: *There is nothing in life that is more predictable than the sheer unpredictability of it.*

*'By releasing the compassion, we can make life more tolerable for carers.'* – Annie Dransfield

# GALLERY

PHOTOS
HOUSES OF PARLIAMENT
HOUSE OF LORDS
CARER AWARDS
ARTICLES

Article: 2012 *Awards Honour our own health service heroes.* NHS Airedale Bradford and Leeds held an event to recognise and celebrate the dedication and commitment shown by members of its Patient Carer and Public Involvement Network, honouring the members who have gone that extra mile. Pride of Airedale Community Champion Award: Annie commended for her efforts in raising carers issues at a national level.

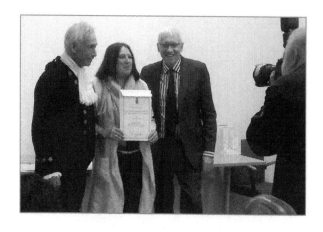

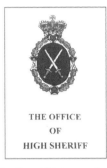 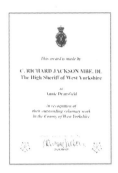

High Sheriff Award: for Banking Campaign

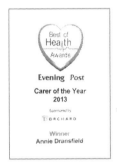

*Yorkshire Evening Post* Best of Health
Carer of the Year Award 2013

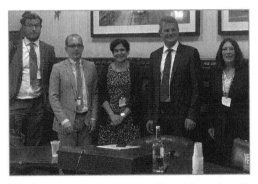

Houses of Parliament Better Banking for Carers –
Meeting with the FCA

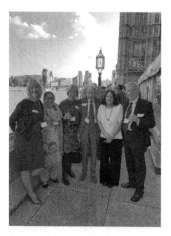

House of Lords

Article: *Carers UK magazine* 2011 Annie, committee member of Carers UK Leeds Branch, cares for her 32-year-old son Jay who suffers from mental health problems and cerebral palsy. Jay has difficulty managing his money so Annie acts as his deputy.

Article: Carers UK Carers and Online Banking.

Article: Carers UK Annie Dransfield Fighting the Banks for Access.

Article: Launching the Leeds Carers Strategy 2015-2018 Annie, Val Hewison, CEO Carers Leeds, and Dame Philippa Russell.

Article: *Yorkshire Evening Post* February 2014. Sarah Freeman interview with Annie on: Families being pushed to the edge as the real cost of caring begins to mount. Carers are the unseen army who save the country millions each year, so why, asks Sarah are there so many carers facing financial crisis?

# REFERENCES

*Business Insider.com Care bots Robobear*

*Business Insider Home and Science*

National Geographic Magazine *the Cities Issue Cities of the Future – fully accessible to the disabled...*

*ArchDaily.com Nicholas Valencia Author of article 'This house was built in 5 days Using recycled plastic'*

*Resumable site Jobs*

*Alianz Care Report Nano Medicine Artificial Intelligence*

*Oxford University – Population Aging*

*Hack and Craft Tokyo's Nursing Home*

*Waypoint Jason Walker Author Robotics*

*Sciencetech Article 5380573B Communicate using thoughts*

*Thrive Gene editing rooms select specific crop variety*

*World Health Organisation How many people will need care in 2050?*

*Digital Empire 2050 65-year-olds outnumber children under 5*

*Alzheimer's Society 850, 00 people in UK*

Mail Online *Zoe Nauman article Humanity will abandon speech and communicate through a collective A1 consciousness using nothing but thoughts by 2050 A1 system HIBA [Hybrid Biometric Avatar] Marko Krajnovic*

*Dana Foundation Author Sophie Fessl, Ph D March 6 2019 Stephen Hawking*

*The* Science Times *Hanna C Aug 28 2020*

*Blog on LSE March 25th 2015 Education*

*Google – Business Insider Collaborative spaces and online platforms*

*Futureeconomics.org Money and Credits in 2050*

*ECO & Beyond Powders and Pills*

*References English Language & Usages Stack Exchange english. stackexchange.com*

*Carers Leeds*

*Carers UK*

*Carers Trust*

*Age UK*

*Adult social services*

www.*AplaceforMom.com*

*Independent Age*

*Alzheimer's Society open access government*

*Digital Empire*

*Population Aging - Oxford University*

*Are Carebots the solution to the elderly care crisis?*

*Hack and Craft*